Working with the Mentally Disordered Offender in the Community

THERAPY IN PRACTICE SERIES

Edited by Jo Campling

This series of books is aimed at 'therapists' concerned with rehabilitation in a very broad sense. The intended audience particularly includes occupational therapists, physiotherapists and speech therapists, but many titles will also be of interest to nurses, psychologists, medical staff, social workers, teachers or voluntary workers. Some volumes are interdisciplinary, others are aimed at one particular profession. All titles will be comprehensive but concise, and practical but with due reference to relevant theory and evidence. They are not research monographs but focus on professional practice, and will be of value to both students and qualified personnel.

1. Occupational Therapy for Children with Disabilities
   Dorothy E. Penso
2. Living Skills for Mentally Handicapped People
   Christine Peck and Chia Swee Hong
3. Rehabilitation of the Older Patient
   Edited by Amanda J. Squires
4. Physiotherapy and the Elderly Patient
   Paul Wagstaff and Davis Coakley
5. Rehabilitation of the Severely Brain-Injured Adult
   Edited by Ian Fussey and Gordon Muir Giles
6. Communication Problems in Elderly People
   Rosemary Gravell
7. Occupational Therapy Practice in Psychiatry
   Linda Finlay
8. Working with Bilingual Language Disability
   Edited by Deirdre M. Duncan
9. Counselling Skills for Health Professionals
   Philip Burnard
10. Teaching Interpersonal Skills
    A handbook of experiential learning for health professionals
    Philip Burnard
11. Occupational Therapy for Stroke Rehabilitation
    Simon B.N. Thompson and Maryanne Morgan
12. Assessing Physically Disabled People at Home
    Kathy Maczka
13. Acute Head Injury
    Practical management in rehabilitation
    Ruth Garner
14. Practical Physiotherapy with Older People
    Lucinda Smyth et al.
15. Keyboard, Graphic and Handwriting Skills
    Helping people with motor disabilities
    Dorothy E. Penso

16. Community Occupational Therapy with Mentally
    Handicapped Adults
    Debbie Isaac
17. Autism
    Professional perspectives and practice
    Edited by Kathryn Ellis
18. Multiple Sclerosis
    Approaches to management
    Edited by Lorraine De Souza
19. Occupational Therapy in Rheumatology
    An holistic approach
    Lynne Sandles
20. Breakdown of Speech
    Causes and remediation
    Nancy R. Milloy
21. Coping with Stress in the Health Professions
    A practical guide
    Philip Burnard
22. Speech and Communication Problems in Psychiatry
    Rosemary Gravell and Jenny France
23. Limb Amputation
    From aetiology to rehabilitation
    Rosalind Ham and Leonard Cotton
24. Management in Occupational Therapy
    Zielfa B. Maslin
25. Rehabilitation in Parkinson's Disease
    Edited by Francis I. Caird
26. Exercise Physiology for Health Professionals
    Stephen R. Bird
27. Therapy for the Burn Patient
    Annette Leveridge
28. Effective Communication Skills for Health Professionals
    Philip Burnard
29. Ageing, Healthy and in Control
    An alternative approach to maintaining the health of older people
    Steve Scrutton
30. The Early Identification of Language Impairment in
    Children
    Edited by James Law
31. An Introduction to Communication Disorders
    Diana Syder
32. Writing for Health Professionals
    A manual for writers
    Philip Burnard
33. Brain Injury Rehabilitation
    A neuro-functional approach
    Jo Clark-Wilson and Gordon Muir Giles
34. Perceptuo-motor Difficulties
    Theory and strategies to help children, adolescents and adults
    Dorothy E. Penso

35. Psychology and Counselling for Health Professionals
   Edited by Rowan Bayne and Paula Nicholson
36. Occupational Therapy for Orthopaedic Conditions
   Dina Penrose
37. Teaching Students in Clinical Settings
   Jackie Stengelhofen
38. Groupwork in Occupational Therapy
   Linda Finlay
39. Elder Abuse
   Concepts, theories and interventions
   Gerald Bennett and Paul Kingston
40. Teamwork in Neurology
   Ruth Nieuwenhuis
41. Eating Disorders
   A guide for professionals
   Simon Thompson
42. Community Mental Health
   Practical approaches to long-term problems
   Steve Morgan
43. Acupuncture in Clinical Practice
   A guide for health professionals
   Nadia Ellis
44. Child Sexual Abuse
   A guide for health professionals
   Celia Doyle
45. Spinal Cord Injury Rehabilitation
   Karen Whalley Hammell
46. Forensic Psychiatry for Health Professionals
   Chris Lloyd

FORTHCOMING TITLES

Motor Neurone Disease
Susan Beresford

Social Skills for People with Learning Difficulties
Mark Burton and Carolyn Kagan, with Pat Clements

Working with the Mentally Disordered Offender in the Community

Phillip J. Vaughan

Park Prewett Hospital,
Basingstoke, UK

and

Douglas Badger

University of Reading,
Reading, UK

CHAPMAN & HALL

London · Glasgow · Weinheim · New York · Tokyo · Melbourne · Madras

Published by Chapman & Hall, 2–6 Boundary Row, London SE1 8HN

Chapman & Hall, 2–6 Boundary Row, London SE1 8HN, UK

Blackie Academic & Professional, Wester Cleddens Road, Bishopbriggs, Glasgow G64 2NZ, UK

Chapman & Hall USA, One Penn Plaza, 41st Floor, New York NY10119, USA

Chapman & Hall Japan, ITP-Japan Kyowa Building, 3F, 2-2-1 Hirakawa-cho, Chiyoda-ku, Tokyo 102, Japan

Chapman & Hall Australia, Thomas Nelson Australia, 102 Dodds Street, South Melbourne, Victoria 3205, Australia

Chapman & Hall India, R. Seshadri, 32 Second Main Road, CIT East, Madras 600 035, India

Distributed in the USA and Canada by Singular Publishing Group Inc., 4284 41st Street, San Diego, California 92105

First edition 1995

© 1995 Phillip J. Vaughan and Douglas Badger

Typeset in 10/12 pt Palatino by Mews Photosetting, Beckenham, Kent
Printed in Great Britain by Page Bros (Norwich) Ltd

ISBN 0 412 56740 7   1 56593 326 5 (USA)

A catalogue record for this book is available from the British Library

Library of Congress Catalog Card Number: 94-69376

Contents

Preface   x
Introduction   xii

1 **Setting the scene**   1
   The basic assumption   1
   Defining the mentally disordered offender   6
   A distinctive way of working   12
   Summary   20
   References   20
   Further reading   21

2 **Policy and legislative framework**   23
   Policy development   23
   Legislation   36
   Summary   45
   References   45
   Further reading   47

3 **Inequality, discrimination and the mentally
   disordered offender**   48
   What is discrimination?   49
   Different forms of discrimination   51
   The power of the worker   54
   The power of the client   56
   How does discrimination happen?   57
   Discrimination against mentally disordered
     offenders   59
   Racial discrimination and the mentally
     disordered offender   64

	Sexual discrimination and the mentally disordered offender	72
	Summary	77
	References	77
4	**The assessment of risk**	**79**
	The human volcano	79
	Risk to others	85
	Risk to the worker	91
	Client's risk to self	98
	Summary	104
	References	105
5	**Primary and secondary prevention**	**107**
	What is primary prevention?	107
	Diversion from custody	114
	Psychiatric/Panel Assessment Schemes	118
	Acting as an 'appropriate adult' under the Police and Criminal Evidence Act 1984	120
	Care management	124
	Probation order with a condition of psychiatric treatment	126
	Supervision and treatment order under the Criminal Procedure (Insanity and Unfitness to Plead) Act 1991	130
	Guardianship orders	131
	The care programme approach	134
	Supervision registers	135
	Summary	137
	References	137
6	**Supervision of patients subject to special restrictions**	**140**
	Work within the hospital setting	140
	Supervision in the community	150
	Summary	168
	References	169
7	**Residential and daycare services**	**171**
	Tasks and functions	173
	Referrals	179
	The ethos	183

Discharge 187
Communication and purpose in residential and
    daycare settings 189
Summary 193
References 194

8   Key issues for the future **195**
Emerging contradictions 195
Training 198
Management support 201
Joint planning and working 203
References 207

**Appendix: The Home Office guidelines on social
    supervision** **209**

Glossary **241**

Index **251**

Preface

In the past forensic psychiatry has been a sub-speciality of general psychiatry without its own, separate identity. However, since the mid-1980s there has been a growing interest in the application of community care principles to mentally disordered offenders. A new set of attitudes have developed which have enabled the mentally disordered offender to emerge from relative institutional obscurity to a much higher profile in the community. Although numerically small in relation to the general psychiatric population, forensic patients tend to attract the public's attention by virtue of their greater propensity for troublesome behaviour. Such a group needs expert community support in order to maintain an acceptable public face.

Unfortunately these developments have outstripped the creation of training opportunities for community staff charged with their support and supervision. Most community practitioners have had to learn 'on the job' with inadequate support and supervision from senior staff, who often have less direct experience of working with this client group than themselves. Just such a situation prompted the authors, in 1990, to establish a module on 'Working with Mentally Disordered Offenders in the Community' as part of an MA in Social Work at the University of Reading. As the course developed it became clear that the topic and content had equal application to other community professionals working in the field.

It also soon became apparent that there was a dearth of published material to refer to, particularly in relation to the practical and ethical issues of working with the offender-patient in the community. Much of the material and case examples therefore were drawn from the authors' and students' own experience. In compiling such material and in developing the emerging themes, this practice handbook was born. The resulting text brings together a wide range of issues that cannot be found anywhere else in the literature. It provides both a practical guide and an operational framework for students, established practitioners and their managers and should appeal to those working in the criminal justice system, mental health services and social services.

We are greatly indebted to students and colleagues whose questions and ideas have stimulated us into writing this book. Appreciation is also expressed to Diane Matthews who patiently and skilfully typed the numerous drafts of the manuscript and to Brian Peters for the artwork. Finally we wish to acknowledge the support and encouragement of our families, especially our wives, who have lived with this book over the past year.

Phillip J. Vaughan and Douglas Badger
June 1994

Introduction

There are three main reasons for writing this book: the time is right, the need is great and there is an absence of literature specifically geared to the busy practitioner trying to make a reality of community care for the mentally disordered offenders. The time is right because today community care is the dominant theme in both health and social services in the UK. For the first time it is a policy that is being extended to mentally disordered offenders and this presents a great opportunity and challenge. On the other hand the closure of the old psychiatric hospitals has led to a lack of secure provision at a local level. The result is that many mentally disordered offenders are being held in prisons or secure units which are not well-suited to their needs. There is a real danger that this group will pay the price for community care for other groups and that they will be the casualties rather than the beneficiaries of the National Health Service and Community Care Act 1990.

The motivation for writing this book arose from the authors' experience of practice with and teaching about this client group. Many of the available publications are written by doctors and psychologists and tend to focus on institutional care. The standard textbooks for community psychiatric nurses and probation officers make little or no reference to this client group and hence provide scant guidance to the practitioner. The existing literature also tends to concentrate on the issues raised by the most serious and dramatic cases. These are often complex and fascinating for both clinical and legal reasons and exert their own hold on the ordinary human curiosity for the macabre and the bizarre. However, the examples discussed are usually far from the everyday experience of most practitioners.

The majority of mentally disordered offenders in the community do not fall into such extreme categories and are far more likely to be described as they were, somewhat uneasily, in the Butler Report (HO and DHSS 1975) as 'inadequates'. The final point about the existing literature is that it is rather scattered, so a major function of this book is to bring together relevant material in a style and a format that makes it readily available.

This book has been written for those who carry professional responsibility for the care and supervision of mentally disordered offenders in the community. It is not specifically addressed to a medical audience, although many of the topics will be of interest to both the psychiatrist and the general practitioner with a commitment to this client group. Identifying precisely which groups the book is written for is difficult when we look further afield than the UK, and even within it there are variations in professional responsibilities and organizational structures. In England and Wales the care and supervision of mentally disordered offenders in the community is a responsibility shared between health, social services and probation in the public sector, and the voluntary, without-profit and profit-making organizations in the private sector. The professional boundaries between those who work in these different settings varies and, for example, in some countries such as Ireland and New Zealand community psychiatric nurses carry many of the duties of an English or Welsh approved social worker. To confuse matters further in many countries, including the UK, responsibility may well be carried by a multidisciplinary team in which roles and functions are shared and can become blurred. In writing a book for such a wide range of staff a recurring difficulty arises about terminology and the generic term of mental health worker will often be employed. However, this is not a description that many probation officers will readily identify with and yet that professional group is highly likely to carry responsiblity for the community supervision of mentally disordered offenders.

More importantly the breadth of the possible readership requires that a wide spectrum of learning needs have to be anticipated, ranging from those of the experienced but possibly untrained manager of a daycentre, through to the recently trained probation officer with little knowledge of mental illness and the psychiatric nurse who is beginning to work in the comumunity, through to the staff of a regional secure unit. Inevitably some parts of the book will be more relevant to some groups of staff and the intention is that the chapter headings and subheadings should help readers to be selective. The working method of the book is that each chapter covers a broad area that is broken down into separate topics. We hope that the busy reader will rapidly be able to identify that part of a chapter which is relevant to a pressing professional concern. For readers such as students who are looking for a more exhaustive treatment it will be more relevant to read an entire chapter.

The structure of the book: Chapter One provides a rationale for a distinctive approach to mentally disordered offenders, looks at definitions of who is to be included in this group, considers the numbers involved and ends with an outline of the elements of a distinctive approach. Chapter Two deals with the British legal and social policy context and provides some history of the treatment of the mentally disordered offender. This should be helpful to all readers but may have particular relevance for those who are new to this field of work or who are comparing the British system with those found in other countries. Chapter Three provides a discussion of discrimination and prejudice in this field. After consideration of the generally unsympathetic light in which mentally disordered offenders are viewed and reported, there is detailed consideration of racial discrimination and a rather briefer discussion of sex discrimination. In each case the factual evidence is reviewed, possible explanations are discussed and implications for practice are drawn out. Chapter Four deals with the assessment of risk and includes a review of the different approaches that have been adopted, including checklists and reliance on procedures. It also pays attention to the impact of this type of work on the staff involved. Chapter Five concentrates on primary and secondary prevention: work that either seeks to prevent those with psychiatric problems from offending or aims to identify those in the criminal justice system whose needs would be better met by the mental health services. The chapter includes case management and divert-to-treatment schemes. Chapter Six deals with the traditional forensic patient: those under restriction orders who are leaving hospital and will be under the care of a social supervisor. The role and statutory responsibilities of the social supervisor are fully described and the whole process from acceptance of the order through transfer to termination is discussed with case material. Chapter Seven covers residential and daycare services and includes discussion of the issues which should be considered at admission, of the match between the ethos and approach of the unit and the needs of the client. The chapter closes with the topic of discharge planning, placement breakdown and staff supervision. Chapter Eight considers likely developments and emerging trends in the field. The book ends with a return to the needs of the worker and to a review of training needs and provision.

Finally, the Home Office guidelines for social supervisors are reproduced as an Appendix, as non-statutory supervisors may not have had the opportunity to see and appreciate the helpful nature of the special supervision arrangements. Additionally, as many of the terms associated with the mentally disordered offender may be unfamiliar to those new to the work, we felt it would be helpful to reproduce in full the glossary of terms used in the Reed Report (Department of Health/Home Office, 1992).

A final point relates to the use of 'he' and 'she' in the text. Wherever possible, generic terms have been used which are not gender specific. However, where this becomes clumsy, 'he' will be used as this is the usual convention. In addition, most mentally disordered offenders are male. In those sections relating specifically to female mentally disordered offenders, 'she' will be used.

REFERENCES

Home Office and Department of Social Security (1975) *Report of the Committee of Mentally Abnormal Offenders*, Cmnd 6244, HMSO, London.

Department of Health/Home Office (1992) *Review of Health and Social Services for Mentally Disordered Offenders and Others Requiring Similar Services*, Cmnd paper 2088, HMSO, London.

1

Setting the scene

The purpose of this chapter is to discuss and hopefully clarify who is included within the term mentally disordered offender and to outline the distinctive approach that is being advocated for those working with this client group. The chapter begins by explaining the basic assumption that there is merit in singling out mentally disordered offenders for special attention. It goes on to identify who might be covered by the term mentally disordered offender and ends with an outline of what is involved in the distinctive approach that is being proposed.

THE BASIC ASSUMPTION

The basic assumption is that mentally disordered offenders have special needs and that it is in their interests and those of the general public that these needs are taken into consideration. This assumption may seem obvious but it is not universally shared and it is important that those working on this assumption are clear in their own thinking. Objections to this approach arise from two primary and very different sources. The first is essentially punitive and sees efforts to divert people from the criminal justice system as examples of interfering do-gooders more interested in the perpetrators of crime than the victims. The other main objection is that offenders who are mentally disordered actually suffer a greater loss of liberty when they are given special consideration than they would have on a straightforward disposal based on the seriousness of their crimes. From this standpoint clients and patients need to be protected from the well-meant but unjust effects of those who seek to help them! To argue against both these objections is to take the position that it is better for the offender, the victim and for society to discriminate between those offenders who are mentally disordered and those who are not.

The term discrimination has now become synonymous with prejudice and disadvantage. This is because it is used as a shorthand for discrimination on unfair or illegal grounds, for example those of race or gender. This limited usage of the word is unfortunate and confusing. It is worth recalling that the term is actually neutral. Indeed, the phrases 'a discriminating eye' and 'a discriminating palate' are usually reserved for someone who is considered to be a good judge of a painting or a wine. In this usage what is being described is the person's ability to assess the strengths and weaknesses of the painting or the wine. This is usually based on experience and knowledge, not qualities commonly associated with the everyday use of the word discrimination! The key to unravelling this conundrum is that both discrimination and assessment require judgement, and all judgements necessarily involve criteria. The crucial question is whether the criteria being used are relevant to the judgement being made. For example, a nursing assessment would be incomplete if it did not include details of the patient's physical health. If it also included details of the patient's political affiliation this would clearly be irrelevant to making a medical or psychiatric diagnosis, and could well lead to the suspicion, if not the reality, of discrimination on political grounds. However, in deciding which candidate to vote for in a General Election it is quite appropriate to consider the candidate's political affiliation as this is a relevant, if not always reliable, criterion in making such a judgement.

The reason for labouring this point about the meaning of discrimination is that the whole premise of this book is that the mentally disordered offender should be treated differently from other people who have committed similar offences. The request to agencies such as the police, the courts and the prison service to treat the mentally disordered offender differently is effectively a request to discriminate between two categories of offenders. This request can only be legal and fair if it is generally accepted that the fact that a person suffers from a mental disorder is relevant to deciding how to deal with their offending behaviour. A recent example shows that even where the judiciary are persuaded that mental disorder is relevant to deciding on a sentence the general public, the police and the relatives of the victim may have another view.

Case study

In July 1993 twenty-six-year-old Paul Gordon was found guilty of the manslaughter of eighty-three-year-old William Horsley, a frail, elderly person with a heart condition. Mr Gordon, who had been diagnosed as suffering from schizophrenia but was refusing medication at the time of the offence, assaulted Mr Horsley and robbed him. Judge Pownall QC took the view that Mr Gordon's diagnosis of schizophrenia indicated that the correct sentence was a three-year probation order with a condition of psychiatric treatment. In making this assessment he presumably took the view that psychiatric illness reduced Mr Gordon's culpability for the offence, and that psychiatric treatment was more likely to reduce the risk of further danger to the public than would a custodial sentence. This judgement proved so controversial that he took the unusual step of recalling all those involved in the case to explain his reasons. Both the victim's niece and the police officer in charge of the case left the court speaking of appeals to the Attorney-General to review the sentence.

(Based on an account in *The Times* 20 July 1993)

This case illustrates a number of dilemmas that arise from arguing that mentally disordered offenders should receive different treatment from others who break the law. The extent to which responsibility is diminished by reason of mental disorder is clearly a matter of judgement and involves some understanding of the nature of different psychiatric diagnoses. In this case most mental health professionals would probably agree in general terms that schizophrenia is a major psychiatric disorder which is likely to impair a person's judgement. This is particularly likely to be true when the person is refusing medication. However, there are significant sections of society that do not share this understanding and this may well

prevent mentally disordered offenders receiving appropriate treatment from groups such as the police and prison
officers. This indicates the crucial importance of education
and training about mental illness for these groups. Much of
the work of divert-to-treatment schemes has this as a key
element.

Even where a shared understanding of mental disorder
exists, there may be dispute about whether the particular
offender has been correctly diagnosed and how disordered that
person was at the time of the offence. In the case study this
was not at issue, but had the diagnosis been psychopathy there
could well have been considerable debate about the general
question of the diagnosis and whether this indicated any
reduction of responsibility for the offence.

The final point relates to the treatability of the condition both in general terms and in relation to a specific
offender. In general terms the symptoms of schizophrenia
can be controlled by the major tranquillizers and specifically Mr Gordon was reported to be responsive to this
medication. As a result it was not difficult to argue for
a community based disposal with a condition of psychiatric treatment. Had psychopathy been the diagnosis there
would have been far more debate about the criteria for
diagnosis and doubt about the likelihood of treatment
being effective. It is also likely that the fact that the treatment would have been social rather than medical might
well have meant that it was viewed with suspicion by the
courts.

In essence, the case for discriminating between mentally
disordered and other offenders rests on the concept of the sick
role and is firmly based on the medical model of mental illness.
This does not invalidate social or psychotherapeutic approaches
but it does assume that these will be adjuncts to rather than
replacements for psychiatric treatments. It is for this reason
that offences related to personality disorder, psychopathy,
alcohol and drug dependency, and sexual deviations which
do not sit comfortably within the medical model cause such
difficulties for the courts and the penal system. Nevertheless
a quasi-medical model is used in relation to these groups
and in so far as individuals are perceived as a) not fully
responsible for their actions, and b) treatable, there is a basis

for arguing that they too should be treated differently from other offenders. However, given the uncertainties that surround both treatability and issues of responsibility, it is not surprising if there are disputes about whether people with these sorts of personality and relationship difficulties should properly be viewed as mentally disordered offenders.

Before concluding this discussion it is important to point out that others in this field take a diametrically opposed position to the one being advocated here. Campbell and Heginbotham (1991) concentrate on the injustices that can be seen to occur when a mentally disordered offender spends a longer time detained in hospital than would have been served in prison as a sentence. They go on to argue that unfair discrimination arises when mental illness is used as a criterion to decide how long a person should lose their liberty rather than the seriousness of the offence. They pursue this argument to its logical conclusion: that mental illness should not be taken into account when considering the disposal of any offender. Though they make the case well it is ultimately unconvincing because it appears to deny any causal link between mental illness and offending behaviour. They also appear to disregard the fact that it is by no means universal that the period spent in hospital exceeds that which might have been spent in prison.

Case study

A young woman, posing as a health visitor, abducted a newly born baby from a London teaching hospital and cared for him for more than a week. The baby was unharmed and returned to his parents. Despite the serious nature of the offence and the media attention it attracted, the offender was sent to hospital for treatment rather than to prison for punishment. She was suffering from depression which responded rapidly to treatment and she was discharged from the regional secure unit within six months. This caused outrage in the popular press as she was seen to be getting off lightly.

DEFINING THE MENTALLY DISORDERED OFFENDER

Having discussed the basic assumption running through the book, the next task is to clarify the term mentally disordered offender. Arriving at a satisfactory definition is not easy because of the difficulties of defining both mental disorder and offending in ways that include those who have not been diagnosed but are suffering from mental illness, and those who are breaking the law but have not been apprehended, charged or convicted. It is, however, possible to identify four groups of mentally disordered offenders whose care in the community currently requires involvement from health and social work staff. These are:

1. those in the community who are suffering from a mental disorder and are committing offences but have not come to the attention of either the criminal justice or the mental health system – the Invisible Mentally Disordered Offenders;
2. those in the criminal justice system who are mentally disordered – Offenders with Mental Health Needs;
3. those in the mental health system whose offending behaviour is not recognized as such – Patients whose Offences are Officially Ignored;
4. those who are or have been in special hospitals, regional and interim secure units, and secure provision in local psychiatric units and hospitals, and those under community disposals such as probation orders with condition of psychiatric treatment – Recognized Mentally Disordered Offenders.

The invisible mentally disordered offender

It is estimated by Goldberg and Huxley (1980) that psychiatric morbidity runs at a rate of about 250 per 1000 population in the community. However, only about 17 per 1000 actually see a psychiatrist and only 6 per 1000 become in-patients in any one year. This means that about 230 persons in every 1000 have a mental health problem which is either receiving no official recognition or is being treated by a general practitioner. How many of these are committing offences is not known and there is no reason to believe that those suffering from mental illness, particularly in its non-psychotic forms, are any more likely to commit offences than the average citizen. However, some of this group may well be receiving some sort of help, care or supervision from social service staff in field, daycare or residential services.

Brown and Harris (1978) in their research on depression in women identified a rate of undiagnosed depression of 17%, and instanced the sorts of processes whereby this comes about. A high-risk group for developing depression were working-class women with three or more children under 14 years, who were not in paid employment and who did not enjoy an intimate relationship with a partner. This group also encountered the most obstacles in getting to a doctor in their own right. Any worker in child protection will recognize such a family unit and may be aware that adult members of that family may have committed offences either against their children or outside the home. However, neither the offences nor the risk of depression may have been fully faced and the implications for effective help and supervision missed by the worker (Cohen and Fisher 1987). A glimpse into the potential seriousness of workers who fail to recognize the potential dangers in this situation is provided by the grim statistic that in the UK a quarter of all murder and manslaughter victims are under 16 years and most are killed by a parent who is mentally ill, especially by the mother (d'Organ, 1979).

Another example can be drawn from residential work with elderly people whose mental health problems may go unrecognized. It might be thought that older people are unlikely to commit offences but in fact there is concern about physical attacks by residents on staff in residential homes. Such incidents are rarely reported to the police and, even if they are reported, the police are encouraged to caution vulnerable people rather than to charge them. As a result the incidents never appear in the criminal statistics. In itself this is not a concern, but the risk is that this will lead staff and others to underestimate the dangers that are involved for themselves and other residents.

In the community, families may also contain 'invisible' mentally disordered offenders – and a mixture of fear and a wish to avoid the stigma associated with mental illness can lead to the containment of such offenders until a serious offence takes place. This is more likely to occur where families do not have good access to medical and psychiatric services, for example when there are cultural and language barriers. The importance of recognizing this group of invisible mentally disordered offenders and responding to their needs is a theme in Chapter Three.

The offender with mental health needs

This group includes those in custody, those under the supervision of probation officers and those who are diverted away from the criminal justice system into psychiatric services. Some attempt will be made to produce figures for these categories but it is worth remembering as a starting point that just as 95% of the public's psychiatric problems are dealt with by general practitioners, so 90% of criminal offences are dealt with by magistrates (Major, 1991) and may not warrant custodial sentences. The majority of offenders are at the lower end of the tariff and may well be sentenced without any consideration of their mental health needs.

The link between mental disorder and offending behaviour is not always clear and different studies reveal rather different pictures. Prins (1980) reviewed a number of small-scale studies and concluded that schizophrenia was numerically insignificant from the point of view of causation or explanation of criminality. However, one of the studies that he reviewed of admissions to Horton Hospital (Rollin, 1969) revealed that of his 78 cases which had not been admitted through the courts 83% had a diagnosis of schizophrenia and 40% had a criminal record, 36% being persistent offenders. More recent British studies tend not to look at this association and figures would anyway be obscured by divert-to-treatment initiatives.

However, a recently reported account of Canadian experience (Webster and Menzies 1993) confirms the view that there is a significant group who move between the criminal justice and mental health systems. The authors followed up two cohorts of people who had been assessed by the Toronto

Forensic Service in 1978 and 1979. For the 571 assessed in 1978 who were followed up two years later, the average length of stay in prison was four months and the average time in hospital was two months. Sixty-one % spent some time in prison and 49% in psychiatric hospital. Twenty-five % spent time in both hospital and prison and only 892 people escaped confinement of one sort or another. The 1979 cohort of 203 people showed a similar profile after two years but this group was also followed up at six years. Of the 195 people traced, 98% had had some sort of contact with the criminal justice or mental health systems. One hundred and fifty-eight people had been imprisoned for an average of 4.4 terms, a total of 11.4 months per person on average. About 50% had had at least one admission to psychiatric hospital and of those admitted the average number of admissions was about three. Only 15 people stayed out of both prison and hospital during the six years. Eighty-one (42%) were in prison only, 22 (11%) were in hospital only and 77 (39%) were in both.

Returning to the scene in the UK, it is not known how many of those on probation orders are disordered but it is safe to assume that the proportion is no less than that in the general population. Pritchard *et al.* (1992) estimate that one fifth will have some sort of mental health problem. This means about two on the average caseload of any probation officer. To what extent their mental disorder contributes to their offending behaviour is not something that can be answered in a global way but it should certainly be part of the assessment of each individual: that is to say, the question should be asked. The number of probation orders with a condition of psychiatric treatment being made is known and the figure for 1991 was 1091. This represents about 2% of all new orders (Hudson *et al.*, 1993).

The prison population of approximately 45 000 convicted and 10 000 unsentenced prisoners undoubtedly includes a proportion of mentally disordered offenders. Wool (1991) notes that the number of remand prisoners who were detainable under the Mental Health Act had changed very little from 1979 to 1987, varying between 150 and 206. The equivalent figures for sentenced prisoners had declined over the same period from 347 to 156, suggesting some success in achieving hospital transfers. The unsentenced population includes 8000 to 9000 people each year who are remanded for psychiatric reports. This is a very high proportion of the remand population and it highlights the difficulties caused by psychiatric hospitals being unable or unwilling to accept the majority of those remanded for psychiatric reports.

Among sentenced prisoners, estimates have varied from as low as 2–3% to 15–20% by Scott (1969). In 1974 Gunn conducted questionnaire research on a sample of 811 men in the prison system and found 31% were considered to be in need of psychiatric treatment. This compares with a figure of 14% in the general population who consult their GP about psychiatric problems in any one year. More recent research by Gunn *et al.* (1991) indicates that between 750 and 1400 sentenced prisoners may currently require transfer to hospital for psychiatric treatment. The discrepancy in the figures probably arises from different criteria being used for mental disorder and variations in the identification of mental illness. With only a third of full-time prison medical officers possessing psychiatric qualifications (Shaw and Sampson, 1991), this would hardly be surprising.

Patients whose offences are not officially recognized

For a number of reasons this group is hard to quantify. The process of diversion has already been cited as obscuring criminal statistics. It has an effect on these statistics too where diversion takes the form of the police not charging an offender but taking them voluntarily or involuntarily to a psychiatric hospital or unit. It is also true that many offences committed by mentally disordered people in mental health settings against other patients, staff or property are not reported or treated as offences and hence fail to emerge in any statistics. This very understandable form of protectionism is not without its risks. It can mean that dangerous behaviour is not recognized as such and this can put people at risk. The inquiry into the death of psychiatric social worker Isobel Schwarz (DHSS, 1988) showed how threats by the patient, Sharon Campbell, were not decisively acted upon. Concern about such condoning of what is actually criminal behaviour has now been translated into guidelines for the safety of staff. Hospital and social services managements are strongly encouraged to make clear their willingness to prosecute clients who threaten staff. This is addressed more fully in the Chapter Four on the assessment of risk.

Perhaps a more useful line of research is to look at those patients who are numerically of most significance to community care staff – the 'revolving door' patients – and to examine whether they have a particular vulnerability to offending. Such research appears not to have been conducted in recent years, possibly because of civil liberties concerns and sensitivities about labelling a group that already carries a heavy burden of stigma. Nevertheless, there is a strong impression that the 'revolving door' patient, particularly if he is homeless, is likely to have a history of petty offending related to vagrancy laws, public order offences, criminal damage and petty theft. Such people will probably come to the attention of probation officers, daycentre staff and hostel workers because of their homelessness. Unless mental health issues are taken into consideration their successful maintenance in the communty is unlikely to be achieved.

Recognized mentally disordered offenders

This group is the easiest to define and count though even it contains a number of people who are not technically offenders because they have not been charged and brought before the courts. However, such patients will usually have created serious management problems within general psychiatric facilities and this effectively is the basis for treating them as offender patients. Hospital order patients may be found in special hospitals, regional and interim secure units, secure and open wards in general psychiatric hospitals, and in the community under supervision. The special hospital population is about 1700 of whom approximately 80% are detained on a court order or following a transfer from prison (Graham, 1991). Approximately 600 mentally disordered offenders can be found in Regional Secure Units and Interim Secure Units, and a further 900 in secure provision within general psychiatric facilities. The number of former patients on restriction orders in the community is between 600 and 700 at any one time.

Summary

This section has advanced a rather inclusive definition of the mentally disordered offender which draws in many such as the troublesome patient and the recurrent petty offender that are often left out of consideration in favour of the restriction order patient. The reason for doing this is that it is thought that those groups can be better catered for if both their mental health needs and their offending behaviour are taken into consideration when work is done with and for them. This implies that for mentally disordered offenders to be successfully maintained in the community, a distinctive approach should be adopted which blends care and control and requires familiarity with both the psychiatric and criminal justice systems.

It is hoped that the discussion of definitions may help non-specialist workers to recognize the mentally disordered offenders with whom they are already working and where necessary to adapt their approach accordingly. The actual numbers involved are hard to establish in any satisfactory way. They appear to be relatively low and this in itself can be a problem as it means that only those working in specialist settings build up the necessary experience and knowledge. On the other hand the widening of the definition of mentally disordered offender brings in many who have not been traditionally identified as mentally disordered offenders and this considerably increases the numbers involved. Those who 'discover' such individuals on their caseloads may take heart from this and realize that they have already accumulated relevant skills in assessment, care and supervision of this client group in the community. Others may find this 'discovery' alarming, but hopefully this book will provide them with some guidance and support.

A DISTINCTIVE WAY OF WORKING

It has been pointed out (Mustill, 1991) that mentally disordered offenders are not an homogeneous group, nor do their 'careers' develop in the same way. Nevertheless they do share certain commonalities, most obviously that they are likely to come to the attention of both the criminal justice and the mental health systems. The proposition being advanced here is that those working with this group also need to develop some commonalities of approach even though their forms of training, professional identities and employing agencies may be very different. The distinctive nature of the approach will be discussed under the headings of Attitudes and Values, Knowledge and Understanding, and Skills.

Attitudes and values

The values and, indeed, the language of community care are centred on concepts such as user, consumer choice, partnership and empowerment. This language does not sit easily with work that may involve the use of statutory powers and acting on behalf of the courts. And yet those under supervision in the community do still retain a lot of choice and autonomy and it would be wrong to view such work as being solely to do with social control. Perhaps the most honest statement is that working with mentally disordered offenders does require co-operation and a sense of partnership but that this can never be an equal partnership. Facing this inequality and disparity in power is an important starting point for anyone who becomes involved with this work.

One approach to thinking about this inequality in power is to reflect on who is the client in any one situation – client in this context being defined as the expected beneficiary of the service provided. In child protection it is clear that this must be the child and that realization helps workers to deal with conflicting responsibilities to parents and to children. In the probation service it is now common (see for example Bryant, 1991) to argue that the community is the client. If the offender is also helped in the process then this is all to the good but the aim is to serve the community by reducing the likelihood of reoffending. Social workers and health workers might have some difficulty in accepting such a formulation as they commonly primarily identify with the task of helping and treating the person in need. However, they too have to be aware of the needs of others and may well intervene to safeguard the health and safety of those members of the community who are in closest contact with the client or patient: the relatives and carers. Both professional groups also become involved in decisions to prevent individuals from committing suicide or harming themselves. This can be seen as a far cry from the philosophy of consumer choice and client self-determination and yet such workers would see themselves as acting in the best interests of the patient or client. This can be understood as acting in partnership with the integrated healthy part of the client's personality to cope with the dangers arising from the disintegrated or disturbed elements of their personalities.

Such an approach can easily be portrayed very negatively in terms of the arrogance of he who knows what is best for others. A more positive understanding is possible if control can be understood as protection and thus as an element in caring rather than as its opposite. This is certainly not the view of extreme libertarians and radical non-interventionists such as Thomas Szasz (1974) who abhor compulsory treatment and defend the individual's right to go mad or commit suicide if he so chooses. However, to be an interventionist does not require an abandonment of the client's right of self-determination but simply a balancing of that right with a duty on others to intervene if somebody is not fully able to judge the situation for themselves. Few rights are absolute and most are balanced by consideration for the rights of others.

The interventionist approach is also informed by an awareness (Irvine, 1979) that if the social control function is not exercised by the community psychiatric nurse, social worker or probation officer then there is every likelihood that it will be exercised by others who would probably do it in a way and a context that would be experienced as harsher and more punitive by the mentally disordered offender. In short, this approach lays far more emphasis on the intervention being appropriate and effective than on the question of whether any intervention should be made at all. While there are obvious dangers of undue intervention, the alternative approach is of intervention being delayed until the situation has become unmanageable and dangerous with the result that agencies such as the police have to become involved. It seems likely that this is at least part of the explanation of why young male Afro-Caribbeans tend to enter the mental health system at the 'heavy end' rather than working up to that only after less intrusive approaches have been tried and failed (Browne, Francis and Crowe, 1993).

Knowledge and understanding

The factual knowledge required is broadly speaking that relating to psychiatry and the mental health system, and the law and criminal justice system. Everyone who has been through professional training will start with some detailed knowledge of their own area of expertise and will only gradually build up knowledge of others areas. This book, for example, should fill some gaps about law and social policy for psychiatric nurses and probation officers. It does not provide detailed knowledge of the court system or the probation service. Such knowledge will best be gained by working with those who do understand that system. There is no substitute for the understanding that will be gained through such experience. Obtaining it may be difficult if there is no tradition of the different disciplines working together or where there has been a history of conflict between key individuals. Current divert-to-treatment initiatives (see Chapter Five) provide a helpful context to those who are looking to gain this knowledge and experience.

Similarly, probation officers may well feel the lack of specific knowledge of psychiatric disorder. Though this book includes some guidance on signs of deterioration, they will not be able to build up a proper knowledge base without further reading and, more importantly, without experience of working with mental health professionals. The presence of local liaison schemes and similar ventures can help in this process but much depends on the attitude of the probation officer and those whom he contacts. For all professional groups there is much to be learned from related disciplines and this understanding of what each has to contribute is essential to good teamwork. In essence, what is needed from all concerned is an understanding and acceptance that safe, effective management of mentally disordered offenders requires a knowledge base that is wider than that of any one of the professional disciplines.

This means that a degree of mutual respect and understanding is not an optional extra but an essential prerequisite. The outcome of such teamwork is an informed understanding of the complex interaction between offending behaviour and mental disorder and an awareness of the full range of possible interventions that may be relevant.

Skills

Making relationships is at the heart of all forms of personal helping and it is the bedrock of working with mentally disordered offenders. It may be that this particular client-group presents more challenges than most in this respect. The worker's own responses to clients who may have committed serious offences is a major concern, as is the importance of being aware of the possibility of being prejudiced against a client-group to whom many are hostile. The clients may also present a challenge in terms of psychological inaccessibility, either because of mental illness or a defensiveness born of frequent exposure to the care system in its widest sense. These then are some of the challenges that the worker may encounter. Yet it is critical that some sort of working alliance is achieved if there is to be any hope of successful care in the community. It is necessary for the client to engage with the task of monitoring his own progress and sharing this with the worker. However comprehensive a care package is arranged, no-one can be with the client 24-hours a day, so establishing this as a shared task between worker and client is very important.

For those who usually rely on their innate capacity to empathize with clients there may also be a challenge. Prins (1986) has warned of the difficulties and dangers of trying to gain too close an understanding of bizarre and unusual behaviour and offences. This was written about those who have committed very serious offences where it is almost impossible for a worker to truly empathize without entering into a world of deeply disturbing thoughts and feelings. However, there are dangers from imagining that one has gained an empathic understanding of all one's clients especially if this is relied on for making predictions of future behaviour.

An acknowledgement that there are limits to the capacity for empathy can be helpful and, if accepted by the worker, can allow a less daunting objective of acceptance of the client and all that he has done coupled with a commitment to fully assessing the client and his offending behaviour.

Prins also makes a strong case for an intrusive style of working for those supervising mentally disordered offenders in the community and though he is particularly addressing the challenge of working with those who have a history of serious offences much of what he has to say is relevant to others. In essence this approach involves a readiness in the worker to insist on entering areas of a client's living and lifespace which conventionally would only occur at the client's invitation. For example, a home visit which might normally be confined to a living-room could well be extended to include the bedroom to check if posters and literature indicated that the client was developing worrying preoccupations or fantasies. Equally, the approach may involve the worker in asking questions about areas of the client's life that are not commonly discussed. Probation officers may be unused to enquiring about disordered thought processes and community psychiatric nurses commonly do not ask about offending behaviour. Learning to check out such matters could well be critical for effective monitoring and supervision of this client group.

It may be helpful to rehearse both the ethics and the practicalities of intrusive casework in individual or group supervision before visiting a client who is giving cause for concern. In effect this is a test of assertiveness and it is important to avoid being so sensitive to the client's feelings that he is unclear what is wanted and why. On the other hand it is also important not to be aggressive and, for example, to demand to see a bedroom in such a way that creates a difficult and potentially dangerous situation.

Important though assertiveness is, it will only get the worker into a position whereby a more thorough assessment can be made. To capitalize on this the worker needs to develop observational and questioning skills. Observational skills may be thought of purely in terms of what is seen but they also involve an ability to keep to the observer role and to put on hold the worker's usual business of helping.

Case study

One of the authors had the experience of visiting the flat of a young male patient after an involuntary admission to hospital. It was the patient's first admission to hospital and it was not very clear whether or not he was mentally ill. He had become obsessed with a young woman at the petrol station where he regularly refuelled his taxi and he began spending many hours in and around the station. She did not welcome his attentions and eventually an order was made forbidding him from approaching the station. He refused to comply with the order and convinced himself that she really did love him. When the police removed him from the premises he rushed into an area where helicopters regularly landed and narrowly escaped being injured or killed.

A home visit was made a few days after the admission to collect some clothes for the patient who by this stage was lucid and apologetic about his behaviour. The flat was chaotic with good quality clothes and equipment strewn around the foor, dirty crockery all over the kitchen and boxes and tins of food covering most surfaces. In the corner of the living room there was a multi-gym and evidence of sporting interests, including a crossbow. The report that was written tried to convey all this to the consultant psychiatrist and ward staff, and the conclusion drawn at the ward round was that it fitted with a male undergraduate lifestyle (the patient had dropped out of university a couple of years previously). The patient was discharged soon afterwards and a home visit revealed some improvement in the state of the flat. A couple of weeks later the patient was readmitted, having attempted suicide with the crossbow. A check on the social work recording revealed that the crossbow had not been included in the report even though the worker had mentioned it several times to colleagues.

Hindsight made clear that the worker had been worried about the crossbow from the start, had made a casual but not intrusive enquiry of the patient about its presence in the flat, and was strangely unsurprised when the patient was readmitted. What had been missing was adequate reflection on what the worker had observed and connection with the dramatic attempt at self-harm which had precipitated the initial admission. This example also illustrates the need to focus on what is being observed and actively to make sense of it. Sometimes there can be a reluctance to think through the possible implications of what is observed. It is not enough to observe keenly: the full implications of what has been seen need to be thought through and faced.

One of the difficulties of an intrusive approach is that it can create a reserve and distance between worker and client. If this happens the worker may well be in danger of losing a crucial ally since it is not realistic to think that supervision in the community can be effective unless the client is engaged at some level in the business of not offending and not breaking down. On the other hand, workers lay themselves open to the charge of gullibility if they do not actively consider the possibility that the client is not sharing everything with them. Though deliberate deception might be the explanation for such behaviour it also needs to be remembered that clients may form strong attachments to workers and they may well feel ashamed and guilty if they have started behaving in an unacceptable way again. In such cases the worker may need help to avoid rejecting the client for letting him down.

This section on skills is not intended to be exhaustive as most, if not all, skills required in working with other client groups are also needed for this group. However, the list would be seriously incomplete if it omitted thoroughness and persistence as essential characteristics of successful workers in this field. To be effective the worker needs to pay attention to detail, from careful perusal of files to listening for discrepancies or oddities in accounts of events. The worker also needs to be persistent, most crucially in relation to the client who may prove elusive, but also in relation to other agencies and professions. It is only too easy for others to forget members of a doubly stigmatized group like mentally disordered offenders. The worker's contribution may be to challenge this inertia on a daily basis by making telephone calls, writing letters and speaking up at case conferences and wardrounds.

SUMMARY

This chapter has outlined the four groups that may be included in any definition of mentally disordered offender and the case was made for an inclusive definition. The numbers involved were outlined and some of the difficulties of obtaining accurate figures discussed. The working assumption that intervention with this client group was needed was then proposed and some of the counter-arguments explored. Finally, a distinctive approach to work in this area was outlined in relation to attitudes and values, knowledge and understanding, and skills.

REFERENCES

Brown, G. and Harris, T. (1978) *Social origins of depression: a study of psychiatric disorder in women*, Tavistock, London.

Brown, D., Francis, E. and Crowe, I. (1993) Black people, mental health and the criminal justice system, in Watson, W. and Grounds, A. *The mentally disordered offender in an era of community care. New directions in provision*, Cambridge University Press, Cambridge, pp. 102–17.

Bryant, M. (1991) *From Client to Clarity – more than a matter of semantics*, Berkshire Probation Service, Reading.

Campbell, T.D. and Heginbotham, C. (1991) *Mental illness: prejudice, discrimination and the law*, Dartmouth, Aldershot.

Cohen, J. and Fisher, M. (1987) Recognition of mental health problems by doctors and social workers. *Practice* 1,(3), 225–40.

Department of Health and Social Security (1988) *Report of the Committee of Inquiry into the Care and After-Care of Miss Sharon Campbell*, Cmnd 440, HMSO, London.

Goldberg, D. and Huxley, P. (1980) *Mental illness in the community*, Tavistock, London.

Graham, C. (1991) A Department of Health perspective, in *The Mentally Disordered Offender*, (eds K. Herbst and J. Gunn), Heinemann, Oxford, pp. 145–55.

Gunn, J., Maden, A. and Swinton, M. (1991) *Mentally Disordered Prisoners*. Home Office, London.

Hudson, B.L., Cullen, R. and Roberts, C. (1993) *Training for work with mentally disordered offenders. Report of a study of the training needs of probation officers and social workers*, CCETSW, London.

Irvine, E.E. (1979) *Social work and human problems. Casework, consultation and other problems*, Pergamon, Oxford.

Major, J. (1991) What can a magistrate do? in *The Mentally Disordered Offender*, (eds K. Herbst and J. Gunn), Heinemann, Oxford, pp. 46–64.

Mustill, M. (1991) Some concluding reflections, in *The Mentally Disordered Offender*, (eds K. Herbst and J. Gunn), Heinemann, Oxford, pp. 225–47.

d'Organ, P.T. (1979) Women who kill their children. *British Journal of Psychiatry*, **134**, 560–71.

Prins, H. (1980) *Offenders, Deviants, or Patients? An introduction to the study of socio-forensic problems*, Tavistock, London.

Prins, H. (1986) *Dangerous behaviour, the law and mental disorder*, Tavistock, London.

Pritchard, C., Cotton, A., Godson, D., Cox, M. and Weeks, S.S. (1992) Mental illness, drug and alcohol abuse and HIV risk behaviour in 214 young adult probation clients. *Social Work and Social Sciences Review*, **3**, (3), 227–42.

Rollin, H. (1969) *The mentally abnormal offender and the law*, Pergamon, London.

Scott, P.D. (1969) Crime and Delinquency. *British Medical Journal* **1**, 424–6.

Shaw, S. and Sampson, A. (1991) Thro' cells of madness: the imprisonment of mentally ill people, in K. Herbst and J. Gunn (eds) *The Mentally Disordered Offender*, Butterworth-Heinemann, Oxford, pp. 104–16.

Szasz, T.S. (1974) *Law, Liberty and Psychiatry*, Routledge & Kegan Paul, London.

Webster, C.D. and Menzies, R.J. (1993) Supervision in the deinstitutionalised community, in *Mental disorder and crime*, (Ed.) S. Hodgkins, Sage, London.

Wool, R.J. (1991) A brief review of the current status of, and provision for, the mentally disordered offender in prison and suggestions for changes, cuts in and research, in K. Herbst and J. Gunn (eds) *The Mentally Disordered Offender*, Butterworth-Heinemann, Oxford, pp. 83–7.

FURTHER READING

Herbst, K.R. and Gunn, J. (eds) 1991 *The mentally disordered offender*, Butterworth-Heinemann, Oxford.

Watson, W. and Grounds, A. (1993) *The mentally disordered offender in an era of community care: New directions in provision*, Cambridge University Press, Cambridge.

2

Policy and legislative framework

Historical background

Community care for the mentally disordered offender is a relatively new concept. Ever since 1482, when it was first established in English common law that it was lawful to incarcerate a dangerous lunatic, either in his own home, or in the local Bridewell, successive government policies and consequent legislation have promoted a custodial approach to this group. It is only in recent years that the inadequacies of custodial institutions, coupled with the drive towards community care policies in general, have brought mentally disordered offenders into consideration as potential recipients of this type of service delivery.

As with non-offender patients, the dangerous and/or offender patient has a long history of custodial care as the only response to the problems they pose, which is well catalogued by Parker (1985). The first specific statutory provision for lunatics was the Vagrancy Act of 1714, which dealt with the 'furiously mad and dangerous' and authorized two or more justices of the peace to have them safely locked up, in chains if necessary. This was followed by the Vagrancy Act of 1744 which introduced the idea of 'curing such person during such restraint'!

However, it was not until 1800 that the first legislative land-mark was reached in relation to the criminal lunatic, in the shape of the Criminal Lunatics Act 1800. This was the outcome of a well-cited incident involving James Hadfield who fired a pistol at George III in Drury Lane theatre in May of that year. Hadfield was found 'not guilty by reason of insanity' but was considered too dangerous to be returned back into the community. To ensure his detention the aforementioned Act was passed and Hadfield was committed to Bethlem Hospital. Under this Act criminal lunatic patients quickly accumulated although there was no specific named place for their detention.

It was not until the County Asylums Act of 1808 that public asylums were required to be built to house all lunatics, including those detained under the Criminal Lunatics Act 1800. At this time medical influences had yet to gain ground and medical certificates for admission and detention had to wait until the advent of the Lunatics Act of 1845. This Act also authorized the continued detention of those who were dangerous and unfit to be at large. Such medical involvement and powers of indefinite detention in hospital still remain with us today.

The next significant landmark was the Criminal Lunatics Act of 1860 which was passed with the purpose of making better provision for the custody and care of criminal lunatics. This led directly to the building of Broadmoor, a purpose-built asylum which opened in 1863. The opening of Rampton in Nottinghamshire eventually followed in 1912. A year later the Mental Deficiency Act 1913 was passed providing comprehensive legislation for mental defectives, resulting in the opening of Moss Side in 1919, for the accommodation of dangerous male defectives. Thus the basis of what was to become the special hospital system was formed.

Just over a decade later developments were to take place within general institutional care for the mentally ill, which were eventually to have an effect on the availability of secure provision within the mental hospital system. The Mental Treatment Act of 1930 introduced the concept of voluntary treatment for the first time. Voluntary patients were free to choose to have treatment and thus encountered a different reception to those who were certified. This extension of boundaries of mental illness and treatment, presumably by increasing the overall numbers in psychiatric hospitals, had the effect of reducing the proportion of the criminally insane among the mental hospital population as a whole. The introduction of the chlorpromazine groups of drugs in the mid-1950s further reduced the need for custody and control which contributed to the consequent reduction of security for psychiatric patients.

However, it was the Mental Health Act of 1959 which had a major impact on the way in which psychiatric services were delivered. It effectively reoriented mental health care away from the institutions and began the process of care in the community.

Local hospitals

Although the Mental Health Act 1959 formed a legal water-shed in relation to custodial hospital care, it was preceded in the early- and mid-1950s by the so-called 'open door' move-ment. The introduction of many positive features into the hospital regime such as occupational and recreational activities, the showing of more respect to patients, improved material benefits, smaller 'groupings' of patients, etc., led in many cases to the removal of any physical restraints over patients in hospital. The doors of wards which had previously been locked were unlocked, allowing patients to come and go as they pleased.

Such developments were heralded as a great success. Patients were reported to be happier and freer, and previous hostility and violence were greatly reduced. Moreover, it was popular with staff. Not surprisingly a belief grew up that physical security must have an adverse effect on patient care and staff morale. There was a feeling that most patients could be contained without physical security with the exception of those difficult or dangerous patients who needed special hospital care. The consequence of this philosophy has been a drastic reduction in the number of locked wards in local NHS hospitals.

Without such secure back-up, difficult patients require high staff ratios to be managed successfully on the ward. Conversely the fewer the staff, the more the anxiety and greater the need to rely on physical methods of restraint. Without high staff ratios or physical barriers, difficult and psychiatric patients abscond. Faulk (1985) presents a well-argued case for retaining

locked wards as a way of meeting the needs of the more
challenging patient. Unfortunately, many people see this as
incompatible with current thinking in terms of psychiatric care:
the use of open hospital wards and domestic style, homely
hostels. In Faulk's view a new culture has developed in local
hospitals. There is a great reluctance to accept difficult patients
and a pool of expertise for managing such inmates has been
lost. Consequently, it has become increasingly difficult to admit
such patients into ordinary psychiatric hospitals. There are
many patients, therefore, who are being denied the benefits
of intensive care in a local mental hospital. Instead there are
patients who Gostin (1985) says are 'sentenced to prison,
inappropriately placed in special hospitals, or simply left in
the community – sometimes sleeping rough, neglected, suicidal
or dangerous'.

Such difficulties were recognized as early as 1959 when the
then Minister of Health warned of the indiscriminate application of the open-door policy. It was realized that some patients
needed adequate security precautions in their own interest and
that of the community. One of the recommendations was that
each hospital maintain some special security precautions. But
alas this did not happen. Such advice was reiterated by the
Department of Health and Social Security in 1971, again to
no avail. More recently the Reed Committee (D of H/HO, 1992)
reported that there should be better access to local intensive
care and locked wards for offender patients in ordinary
psychiatric provision. The report further stated that 'the
number of beds in locked or lockable wards fell from 1163 for
mental illness and 785 for learning disabilities in 1986 to 639
and 274 respectively in 1991'.

With the mental hospital closure programme now well
under way the situation can only deteriorate further, as the
small acute units that are replacing the large asylums have little
capacity for secure provision.

The prison system

The above changes, particularly the loss of asylums post-1959,
have swelled the psychiatric population within the prison
system. Hospital managers have the discretion to refuse the
admission of any patient, with the result that judges cannot

compel a hospital to admit a mentally disordered offender on sentence. Prison governors, on the other hand, have no such discretion and have to accept any person sent to them by the court. As it is often difficult to find a suitable hospital bed, many people who need psychiatric care inappropriately end up in custody.

The actual number of prisoners requiring mental health care is not known but it is thought that 2%–3% of sentenced prisoners have a psychiatric illness and that a greater percentage is to be found among the remand population. Increasing numbers of prisoners are also found to be suffering from drug and alcohol abuse, personality disorder and neurotic illnesses. Recent research by Gunn *et al.* (1991) suggests that between 750 and 1400 sentenced prisoners may currently require transfer to hospital for psychiatric treatment.

Furthermore, there is evidence of courts remanding the mentally disordered for psychological and social reasons rather than for public safety reasons or because of the seriousness of the offence. In many instances the prison system is clearly being wrongly used. There are between 8000 and 9000 remands to prison per annum solely for psychiatric reports, which severely aggravates the situation. This group who present with symptoms of mental abnormality could be more suitably remanded to hospitals or clinics. As mentioned previously, however, NHS hospitals no longer have the stomach or capacity for secure care, leaving the courts no option but to remand such people to prison.

The situation is well-illustrated by the decrease in the number of mentally disordered offenders who were transferred from prison, for treatment in hospital between 1961 and 1976. In 1961, 179 sentenced men were transferred from prison to hospital, whereas by 1976 this figure had declined to only 30 (Gunn, 1985).

Interestingly, despite the obvious need for psychiatric care within the prison system, the prison medical service is not and has never been part of the National Health Service. Resources for offering prisoners proper psychiatric care and treatment are scarce. Apart from its one specialized psychiatric prison, Grandon Underwood, the system depends largely on visiting psychiatrists and psychotherapists. With no significant expansion of psychiatric services in prisons being planned and with a persistently high prison population, the situation is unlikely to improve in the foreseeable future.

The special hospitals

The special hospital system was created as a result of Section 97 of the Mental Health Act 1959, later repealed and replaced by Section 4 of the National Health Service Act 1977. It required the Secretary of State for Social Services to provide special hospitals for 'detained mentally disordered patients, who in his opinion, require treatment under conditions of special security on account of their dangerous, violent or criminal propensities'. As a result, Broadmoor, Rampton and Moss Side were designated for this purpose in 1959 and were managed directly by the Department of Health. In 1974 a new special hospital, Park Lane, was opened and in 1989 was merged with Moss Side to become known as Ashworth.

In 1989 responsibility for the special hospitals was transferred from the Department of Health to the newly created Special Hospitals Service Authority which has the following aims:

1. to ensure the continuing safety of the public;
2. to ensure the provision of appropriate treatment for patients;
3. to ensure a good quality of life for patients and staff;
4. to develop the hospitals as centres of excellence for the training of staff of all disciplines in forensic and other branches of psychiatric care and treatment;
5. to develop close links with the NHS local and regional psychiatric services;
6. to promote research into fields related to forensic psychiatry.

Nevertheless, despite these laudable aims the special hospitals remain marginalized from the mainstream psychiatric services. Unlike the clientèle of the 'open-door' hospitals all patients in special hospitals are detained, mostly under provisions of the Mental Health Act 1983. Such patients are regarded as presenting a grave danger to the public and to require the highest level of security. This puts the special hospitals at the far end of the security/treatment spectrum which presents its own problems. As with any other treatment setting, these hospitals can only operate effectively if they are seen as part of an integrated system of care and treatment. That means co-operation with and movements between other institutional and community services. While patients are clearly in need of treatment under conditions of special security when they are admitted to a special hospital, many respond to treatment, are stabilized and eventually need discharge. Herein lies the rub. Having been tainted by the label of being a special hospital patient, inmates face the problems of stigma and prejudice which often blocks their subsequent access to community facilities. Conventional psychiatric hospitals are not keen to take such patients and community hostels are equally wary, if not unsuitable as a first step towards community integration for the ex-special hospital patient. Not surprisingly, a census by the Special Hospitals Service Authority revealed that approximately 400 patients currently in special hospitals may not require the highest levels of security and should be transferred to regional and local secure services (SHSA, 1991).

Gostin (1985) goes as far as to claim that: 'It is unlawful and harmful to a patient's prospects for treatment and rehabilitation, for him to remain in conditions of security longer than is necessary'. He goes on to quote similar statistics to illustrate the rising lengths of the waiting list for transfer and discharge.

Although, therefore, special hospitals offer virtually the only long-term secure treatment settings, their uniqueness is potentially isolating and more bridges are needed to link them to mainstream services.

Regional secure units

It will be clear from the above that there is an enormous gap between the open-door provision of most local hospitals and that of the high security afforded by the special hospitals. There are many patients whose difficult behaviour exceeds the capacity of staff working on an open ward and yet is not sufficiently dangerous to warrant incarceration in conditions of high security. Such problems were first recognized as long ago as 1961 when the Ministry of Health welcomed the development of the open-door movement but concluded that secure accommodation should be retained by National Health

Service hospitals for those patients who needed it. It was recommended that some designated secure units be set up along with special diagnostic treatment and assessment centres. Such developments, however, did not occur and it was not until the mid-1970s that the situation was examined again in any detail.

In 1974 the Glancy Report was published (DHSS, 1974) which expressed concern about the virtual absence of security arrangements in the Regional Health Authorities, and recommended that each provide an initial total of 1000 secure beds for England and Wales. Meanwhile the Butler Committee had been established in 1972 and was focusing its attention on, among other things, the lack of secure provision specifically for the mentally abnormal offender. Its interim report published in 1974 (HO and DHSS, 1974) recognized the huge gap between the secure provision of the special hospitals and the open-door provision of the NHS hospitals. Accordingly it strongly recommended the building of regional secure units to bridge this gap. An initial target of 1000 secure places was suggested, with further increases of up to 2000 secure places if required, to be funded by central government.

The final report was presented in 1975 (HO and DHSS, 1975) and had the effect of pumping money and political influence into forensic services. Disappointingly, however, despite the early enthusiasm from central government, the Regional Health Authorities were slow to act and it was not until 1980 that the first Regional Secure Unit was opened. Even by 1992 only approximately 600 beds had been established, far short of the target of 1000 (D of H/HO, 1992). It is hoped that this number will be achieved by 1995, with increased capital funding announced in 1992 of £18 million.

Unfortunately the creation of the RSUs has not entirely solved the problem. As the number of long-stay psychiatric beds decrease, those 'difficult' patients needing asylum are being referred to the RSUs in the absence of any other suitable resource. It was intended that RSUs keep patients for no longer than two years, preferably eighteen months, in order to maintain some movement through the system. Increased pressure to take longer-term patient simply clogs up the system and makes it more difficult for medium-secure facilities to serve the special hospitals and prisons as intended.

Unfortunately such deficiencies often result in the mentally disordered offender ending up in the community by default as illustrated by Mr. H.:

Case study

Mr. H., a 23-year-old single man, was remanded to prison for psychiatric reports, following a relatively minor offence. He was clearly suffering from a mental disorder and a consultant psychiatrist recommended admission to hospital under Section 3 of the Mental Health Act 1983. The consultant also stated that Mr H. was unsuitable for an open ward and needed to be admitted to secure accommodation. However, as there was no medium-secure bed available and the general psychiatric hospital refused to accept him the application was not pursued. The police, meanwhile, being unable to detain Mr H. further, had no option but to discharge him back into the community.

Home Office circular no. 66/90

The Home Office circular No. 66/90 was dated 3 September 1990 and was targeted at the Criminal Justice System and associated services and personnel responsible for dealing with mentally disordered persons who commit, or who are suspected of committing, criminal offences (Home Office, 1990). The clearly stated government policy is that the mentally disordered should receive care and treatment from Health and Social Services wherever possible in preference to formal prosecution. Accordingly alternative measures should always be considered first, such as the use of caution, hospital care and treatment or support in the community. In order to achieve these aims, consultation and co-operation is required between health authority, social services departments and the judiciary.

More specific guidelines are issued to the key players in the criminal justice system:

Police: the agency of first contact is reminded of its powers to use Sections 135 and 136 of the Mental Health Act 1983. Where an offence is suspected to have been committed then a caution can be used or a diversion from the criminal justice system effected by accessing the relevant sections of the Mental Health Act 1983 or by providing support in the community. Where prosecution is necessary, bail in a hostel or hospital should be used where possible on a voluntary basis. After a mentally disordered person has been charged an assessment should be made to ensure medical treatment is provided as necessary.

Crown Prosecution Service: where the probable effect upon the person's mental health outweighs the interests of justice, the CPS should consider discontinuing the proceedings.

Magistrates Court/Crown Court: a mentally disordered person should not be remanded to prison simply to receive medical treatment or assessment. Professional advice should be obtained as early as possible. Non-penal disposal should be sought where possible including the use of the appropriate sections of the Mental Health Act 1983. A probation order with a condition of psychiatric treatment should also be considered where suitable.

Probation Service: the probation officer's role in networking and liaison with community agencies is highlighted, as is the importance of establishing links with bail hostels and other forms of accommodation.

Prison Medical Service: prison medical officers are reminded of the need to be alert for signs of mental disorder and to recommend transfer to hospital where necessary.

In retrospect 1990 may be seen as a watershed in the government's approach to working with the mentally disordered offender. The promotion of diversion and discontinuance mechanisms to avoid unnecessary involvement with the Criminal Justice System may be seen as an important step in reversing the pointless criminalization of this group of people. Nevertheless, the success of such schemes depend on energetic inter-agency co-operation and perhaps even more importantly adequate funding to provide the range and volume of community services necessary. NACRO highlights the competing demands on limited service by other user groups, particularly the elderly, following the implementation of the NHS and Community Care Act 1990 in April 1993. It quotes an estimate of a £54m shortfall in terms of maintaining existing community support services and a possible £289 million shortfall in the total proposed allocation of funding (NACRO, 1993). The community care of mentally disordered offenders may not feature highly in the consequent pressure to restrain expenditure.

Without such financial support, diversion and discontinuance schemes are likely to be curtailed.

The Reed report 1992

The Reed Report is the most important and far-reaching review of health and social services for mentally disordered offenders since the Butler Report of 1975. Established by the Department of Health and the Home Office under the Chairmanship of Dr John Reed, the committee met for the first time on 31 January 1991 and completed its work on 23 July 1992. The final report was published in November 1992. Its guiding principles were that patients should be cared for:

1. with regard to the quality of care and proper attention to the needs of individuals;
2. as far as possible, in the community, rather than in institutional settings;
3. under conditions of no greater security than is justified by the degree of danger they present to themselves or others;
4. in such a way as to maximize rehabilitation and their chances of sustaining an independent life;
5. as near as possible to their own homes or families if they have them.

The final report (D of H/HO, 1992) contains no less than 276 recommendations addressing the following key issues:

- a positive approach to the needs of individual patients, many of whom including women and people from ethnic minorities, may have special or differing needs;
- a flexible and multi-agency approach whose aim is to identify and meet most effectively the needs of mentally disordered offenders;
- closer working between the police health and social services to avoid unnecessary prosecution of mentally disordered suspects;
- the development of the probation service to
  1. facilitate effective co-operation at local level between criminal justice agencies and health and social services
  2. ensure that prosecutions are not initiated where they could be avoided and

    3. help divert from custodial disposals mentally disordered people who have to be prosecuted;

- an improved range of community care services, including accommodation and day services that are suitable as alternatives to prosecution and will meet the needs of homeless mentally disordered offenders;
- the expansion of medium secure and 'outreach' services, including in particular those to cater for people with learning disabilities and longer-term medium security needs;
- the improvement of mental health services for prisoners, to be contracted in mainly from the NHS;
- a stronger academic and research base to underpin service improvements and the general and specialized forensic training of staff to work with mentally disordered offenders.

The resource implications of the review are considerable and although it states that much could be achieved through better co-ordination and more effective use of resources it also makes clear that substantial service development cannot be made within existing resources. Unfortunately, this was not a view shared at its launch by the then junior health minister, Tim Yeo, who said that progress in the care and treatment of mentally disordered offenders could be achieved by 'better use of existing services and resources'.

    It would be sad indeed if such an important review was stymied at the outset by lack of government funding. How many of the 276 recommendations are implemented remains to be seen.

The Care Programme Approach

The Care Programme Approach which was introduced in the NHS in April 1991, followed the issuing of a joint Health and Social Services Circular in 1990 (D of H, 1990). It required district health authorities in collaboration with local social services departments to set up individually tailored care programmes for all in-patients about to be discharged from mental illness hospitals and all new patients accepted by the specialist psychiatric services.

    The Care Programme Approach involves a systematic assessment of the health and social care needs of the patients, the drawing up of a package of care agreed by the multidisciplinary team, patient and carer, the nomination of a key worker and regular review and monitoring of the patient's needs and progress.

Although there are some similarities with the care management process, the Care Programme Approach is complementary to it. Indeed, the key worker role under the Care Programme Approach and the role of the care manager in care management are distinct. Generally speaking the key worker will have some responsibility for service delivery but no budgetary control, whereas the care manager will control the budgetary requirements of the care package and act as a broker for services across the statutory and independent sectors.

This additional process provides another safety net for mentally disordered offenders as well as psychiatric patients generally to ensure that in future all patients treated in the community receive the health and social care they need.

Supervision register

From 1 April 1994 all health service provider units providing mental health care, were required to 'set up registers which identify and provide information on patients who are, or are liable to be at risk of committing serious violence or suicide, or of serious self-neglect, whether existing patients or newly accepted by the secondary psychiatric services' (NHS Management Executive, 1994). The stated purpose of the register is to ensure that those who pose most risk in the community receive adequate care, support and supervision. Many mentally disordered offenders are prime candidates for such registers, although registration on its own does not guarantee that the appropriate resources will be made available. Nevertheless, the intention is that those on the register should receive the highest priority of care and active follow-up. A fuller discussion of the register's application is found in Chapter Five.

Without doubt the needs of the mentally disordered offender have received a much higher profile in recent years and forensic psychiatry has emerged as a speciality in its own right. Table 2.1 illustrates the chronological development of government policies and legislation affecting this group. However, without additional funding to support the latter initiatives, community services will continue to be slow to develop.

Table 2.1 Chronology of policies and legislation impacting on the care and treatment of the mentally disordered offender

1482	Under English Common Law dangerous lunatics could be incarcerated
1714	Vagrancy Act
1744	Vagrancy Act
1800	Criminal Lunatics Act
1808	County Asylums Act
1845	Lunatics Act
1860	Criminal Lunatics Act
1863	Broadmoor Opened
1912	Rampton Opened
1913	Mental Deficiency Act
1919	Moss Side Opened
1930	Mental Treatment Act
1959	Mental Health Act
1974	Park Lane Opened
1974	Glancy Report
1975	Butler Report
1983	Mental Health Act
1984	Police and Criminal Evidence Act
1989	Special Hospitals Service Authority established
1989	Ashworth Opened
1990	Home Office Circular 66/90
1990	National Health Service and Community Care Act
1991	Criminal Procedure (Insanity and Unfitness to Plead) Act
1991	Criminal Justice Act
1991	Care Programme Approach Introduced
1992	Reed Report
1994	Supervision Registers Introduced

LEGISLATION

The central legislative tool used in connection with the mentally disordered offender is Part III of the Mental Health Act 1983 supplemented by a few other relevant pieces of legislation. It is not intended to describe each piece of legislation in detail, as comprehensive texts are readily available on mental health law. Nevertheless, it is useful to summarize the legal framework within which mental health practitioners have to operate in relation to compulsory detention.

Mental Health Act 1983

Part II of the Act provides for the detention of 'civil' patients in hospitals or mental nursing homes for the medical treatment of mental disorder. Offender patients may also be treated under this part of the Act, particularly as a result of being 'diverted to treatment' as part of a Division Scheme. The relevant sections include:

Section 2: admission for assessment (perhaps followed by medical treatment) for a maximum of 28 days;

Section 3: admission for treatment for a maximum of six months;

Section 4: emergency admission for a maximum period of 72 hours;

Section 5: detention of a patient already receiving treatment in hospital on an informal basis, for a maximum period of 72 hours;

Section 7: applications for Guardianship;

Section 136: authorizes a police constable to remove from a public place, a person who appears to be suffering from mental disorder and to be in immediate need of care and control, to a place of safety for examination for a maximum period of 72 hours;

Part III of the Act contains the bulk of the sections relevant to the mentally disordered offender, viz:

Section 35: (remand to hospital for a report) A Crown Court or magistrate's court can remand an accused person to a specified hospital for a report to be obtained on his mental condition;

Section 36: (remand to hospital for treatment) As an alternative to remand in custody, the Crown Court may remand an accused to hospital if satisfied on evidence of two doctors, that the accused is suffering from mental illness or severe mental impairment which makes it appropriate for him to be detained in hospital for medical treatment;

Section 38: (Interim hospital order) A Crown Court or magistrate's court may send a convicted offender to hospital for up to six months to enable an assessment to be made as to the appropriateness of making a hospital order;

Section 37: (Hospital order) The Crown Court or Magistrate's Court where a person has been convicted of an offence, punishable with imprisonment, may authorize detention in hospital or guardianship provided that all the appropriate criteria for such an order are met;

Section 41: (Restriction Order) A Crown Court (or the Court of appeal) may make a restriction order when it decides to place an offender on a hospital order, if it appears to the court that it is necessary to protect the public from serious harm. Such an order may impose special restrictions either without limit of time or during such period as may be specified in the order;

Section 47: (Transfer from prison to hospital of a sentenced prisoner) The Home Secretary may transfer a sentenced prisoner to a hospital (not a nursing home) so that he may be detained for medical treatment.

Section 48: (Transfer of other prisoners from prison to hospital) Prisoners other than those serving a sentence may be transferred to hospital from prison by the Home Secretary if he considers it appropriate, e.g. prisoner on remand.

Readers who require a more detailed description and analysis of the workings of the Mental Health Act 1983 are referred to the comprehensive text *The Law of Mental Health* (Williams, 1990).

Police and Criminal Evidence Act 1984 (Section 66)

The original Codes of Practice for the above Act were introduced in January 1986 and revised with effect from 1 April 1991 (Home Office, 1991). Annexe E to Code C summarizes the provision relating to mentally disordered and mentally handicapped persons.

It states that if a police officer suspects, or is told in good faith, that a person is suffering from a mental disorder or is mentally handicapped, or mentally incapable of understanding the significance of questions put to her/ him, then that person shall be treated as a mentally disordered or mentally handicapped person for the purposes of the code.

It goes on to say that although such persons are often capable of providing reliable evidence, they may, without knowing or wishing to do so, be particularly prone in certain circumstances to provide information which is unreliable, misleading or self-incriminating. Special care should therefore always be exercised in questioning such a person, and an appropriate adult should be involved if there is any doubt about a person's mental state or capacity.

Accordingly a person who is mentally disordered or mentally handicapped, whether suspected or not, must not be interviewed or asked to sign a written statement in the absence of an appropriate adult unless there is a need for an urgent interview. (See Annex C).

The role of the appropriate adult is to:

1. advise the person being questioned;
2. observe whether or not the interview is being conducted properly and fairly; and
3. to facilitate communication with the person being interviewed.

A fuller discussion of the role of the responsible adult can be found in Chapter Five.

National Health Service and Community Care Act 1990

The above Act, which was finally fully implemented on 1 April 1993, represents a significant change in the delivery of health and social care services. The 1989 White Paper (D of H, 1989), which preceded it, provided a description of the intended impact of the Act and stated that the central objective of community care is to enable people to: 'Live as normal a life as possible in their own home or in a homely environment in the local community'.

The White Paper also identified the four key components of the new style community care which underpin the changes. These are services:

1. that respond flexibly and sensitively to the needs of individuals and carers;
2. that intervene no more than is necessary to foster independence;
3. that allow a range of options for consumers; and
4. that concentrate on those with the greatest need.

Local authorities become the lead agency in answering individual need and arranging 'packages of care'. Each recipient of service has a care manager whose task it is to implement, co-ordinate, monitor and review that care package. Potentially this has great benefits for the mentally disordered offender.

Interestingly such developments evolved from mental health care in North America where care management was introduced as a response to poor inter-agency collaboration. Although the Community Mental Health Centre Act of 1963 lead to an increase in the range and quality of community services, it was found that those with a serious mental illness had difficulty in accessing them and were regularly falling through the net of caring agencies. Care management was specifically designed to help those with severe and long-term mental health problems.

Until now mentally disordered offenders have had the potential of being the worse served, particularly those who commit petty offences. Unfortunately they are not always a popular or easy group to help and agencies will often avoid responsibility for their care and treatment. Accordingly there is much experience of mentally disordered offenders committing nuisance offences simply to obtain shelter, warmth and food. The introduction of care management should ensure that this group of offenders get a better response from the statutory agencies. However, much will still depend on good collaboration between them – and to date this has not always been good.

Another potential problem in the health and social care divide is described by Onyett (1992). The mentally disordered offender has needs that often straddle the boundaries between health and social care, causing each agency to look to the other for the funding of services. Onyett also warns of future funding shortages hampering service development and tightening the criteria for intervention. Indeed, mental health care is already the Cinderella of local authority provision with most authorities allocating a mere 4% of their total care budget for this group. Mentally disordered offenders are the Cinderella of mental health care and even with the introduction of care management will find it difficult to compete for adequate resources in the face of so many other demands on services.

Criminal Procedure
(insanity and unfitness to plead) Act 1991

The above Act, which replaced the Criminal Procedure (Insanity) Act 1964, was implemented on 1 January 1992 and has the following features:

A trial of the facts: Where an accused person has been found unfit to be tried, there is provision for there to be a 'trial of the facts' to determine whether the accused did the act or made the omission charged against him. If the court is satisfied that this is the case it will make a finding to that effect; such a finding is not the equivalent of a conviction.

Medical Evidence: A jury is not to return a verdict of not guilty by reason of insanity under the Trial of Lunatics Act 1883 except on the evidence of two or more medical practitioners, at least one of whom is duly approved by the Secretary of State under Section 12 Mental Health Act 1983.

Disposal options: Where the accused has been found unfit to be tried (and following a trial of the facts, to have done the act or made the omissions charged against him) or not guilty by reason of insanity, the court is able to choose between a range of options, i.e.:

Hospital order: an order for detention in such hospital as the Secretary of State might direct may be made by the court. In addition, a restriction order without limit of time will be imposed when the offence charged is one for which the sentence is fixed by law (i.e. murder). In other cases the court retains the option to impose a Restriction Order for a specified period or without limit of time.

Guardianship Order: a guardianship order may be made under the provisions of Section 37 of the Mental Health Act 1983. The purpose of the guardianship order is primarily to ensure that the offender receives care and protection rather than medical treatment, although the guardian does have powers to require the offender to attend for medical treatment.

Supervision and Treatment Order: this order is modelled on a probation order with a condition of psychiatric treatment. It requires the offender to be under the supervision of a social worker or a probation officer for a period to be specified in the order, not exceeding two years.

Absolute Discharge: this option may be considered where the alleged offence was trivial and the offender does not require treatment and supervision in the community.

Criminal Justice Act 1991

The above Act affects mentally disordered offenders in the following areas:

Sentencing

To allow the court to form an opinion as to whether the offence justifies a custodial sentence a pre-sentence report should be obtained unless the offender is convicted of an indictable only offence and the court thinks it unnecessary. If therefore the offender is or appears to be mentally disordered the court shall obtain and consider a medical report before passing a custodial sentence. However, there is no such requirement in the case of an offence fixed by law or if the court is of the opinion that it is 'unnecessary' to obtain a report.

Before passing a custodial sentence on a person who is considered to be mentally disordered the court must consider any information which relates to the person's mental condition and the likely effect of such a sentence on that condition and on any treatment that may be available.

Information concerning guardianship

Section 27 of the Criminal Justice Act 1991 amends Section 39 of the Mental Health Act 1983. Now, a court considering making a guardianship order in respect of any offender may require the appropriate local authority to inform the court whether it, or any other person approved by it, is willing to receive the offender into guardianship. If this is the case, the local authority should give such information as it reasonably can about how it or the other person could be expected to exercise its powers in relation to guardianship.

Reduction of period for making hospital orders

Section 37 of the Criminal Justice Act 1991 amends Section 37 of the Mental Health Act 1983. Where a court makes a hospital order, or interim hospital order, the time limit for admission may now be reduced from 28 days.

Early release of prisoners

Most persons transferred from prison to hospital are subject to a 'restriction direction', which ceases on expiration of the person's sentence. The concept of remission is now abolished and superseded by an automatic release provision. Section 50 (3) of the Mental Health Act 1983 is amended to remove any reference to remission.

Probation order with a condition of psychiatric treatment

With the development of child guidance clinics in the 1920s and psychiatric out-patients clinics in the 1930s, some influential London magistrates began to insert conditions of psychiatric treatment in probation orders. This practice received statutory recognition under the Criminal Justice Act 1948. Such orders were originally for one year and were extended to three years by the Criminal Justice Act 1972 and subsequently by the Powers of Criminals Courts Act 1973, as amended by the Criminal Justice Act 1991.

Essentially this is a normal probation order which requires the consent of the offender. It is adapted to meet the needs of the offender who does not need detention but who has a mental health condition which can be treated. Accordingly the offender is required to undertake treatment for the whole or part of the order under one of the following conditions:

1. residential treatment at a specified hospital;
2. non-residential treatment at a specified place;
3. treatment by or as directed by a named doctor.

The key to the success of such orders appears to be the careful selection of suitable offenders, clarity of roles between the probation officer and psychiatrist and good co-ordination between the services involved (Lewis, 1980; Walker, 1985).

Proposed supervised discharge arrangements

In recent years there has been increasing disquiet over the plight of the mentally ill in the community. Concern has been felt about many seriously ill patients who have been discharged from hospital without adequate after-care or have refused to comply with the after-care arrangements that have been made. There are a small number of people mostly with a diagnosis of schizophrenia who persistently avoid contact with the statutory mental health agencies. In doing so they fail to maintain their regime of prescribed medication, are regularly non-attenders at out-patient clinics and frequently have chaotic lifestyles. Inevitably their mental health deteriorates, often to the extent that they become a risk to themselves or others. It is not until a crisis occurs that they are apprehended and re-admitted to hospital, usually under a section of the Mental Health Act 1983.

A number of tragedies in the early 1990s involving people suffering from schizophrenia led the government to review the options for supervising disturbed patients in the community (D of H, 1993). Despite a strong bid by the Royal College of Psychiatrists to introduce a Community Supervision Order (Royal College of Psychiatrists, 1993) the Department of Health decided against such a measure, opting instead for some modifications to existing procedures. It also proposed to amend the Mental Health Act 1993 to provide for 'the supervised discharge of non-restricted patients who have been detained in hospital under the Act and who would present a serious risk to their own health or safety, or to the safety of other people, unless their care was supervised'.

The proposed supervised discharge arrangements embody the principles of the Care Programme Approach together with the key features of guardianship. However, there is some scepticism about the usefulness of such a measure, particularly as the guardianship which it closely resembles has been largely ineffective. Bluglass (1993) takes the view that 'These recommendations are a compromise solution that reflects the lack of consensus among users, carers and professionals about tackling this difficult group of patients.' Only experience will show how effective such measures will be.

SUMMARY

Social policy and legislation in relation to the mentally disordered offender have been historically linked to institutional care. Whereas community care policies and practice for general psychiatry were triggered by the Mental Health Act 1959, forensic psychiatry had to wait a further 30 years before being influenced by the community care movement.

Meanwhile, NHS psychiatric provision for this group diminished considerably during this period and the prison service continued to absorb increasing numbers of inmates with psychiatric problems. It was not until 1990, however, that there was any definitive statement from the government about its intentions for community based care for offender-patients in the shape of Home Office circular 66/90 (Home Office, 1990). This circular, along with the publication of the Reed Report (D of H/HO, 1992), spearheaded the way for developing community services for this group.

Diversion schemes have realigned response patterns to mentally disordered offenders presenting to the criminal justice system, particularly for those who commit relatively minor or 'nuisance' offences. However, although their needs have been more appropriately redirected, policy developments have yet to produce additional resources to meet them.

The establishment of supervision registers for vulnerable at-risk patients in the community, and the proposed supervised discharge arrangements for non-compliant potentially dangerous patients leaving hospital, have introduced elements of authority and control into community based work which has hitherto been absent among those patients not subject to a court order.

REFERENCES

Bluglass, R. (1993) New powers of supervised discharge of mentally ill people. *British Medical Journal*, Vol. 307, 6 November, 1160.

Department of Health (1989) *Caring for People: Community Care in the Next Decade and Beyond*, HMSO, London.

Department of Health (1990) *The Care Programme Approach for People with a Mental Illness Referred to the Specialist Psychiatric Services*, HC (90) 23, LASSL (90), II, Department of Health, London.

Department of Health (1993) *Legal Powers on the Care of Mentally Ill People in the Community*, Report of the Internal Review, Department of Health, London.

Department of Health/Home Office (1992) *Review of Health and Social Services for Mentally Disordered Offenders and Others requiring Similar Services*, Final Summary Report Cmnd 2088, HMSO, London.

Department of Health and Social Security (1974) *Revised Report of the Working Party on Security in NHS Psychiatric Hospitals*, (The Glancy Report), DHSS, London.

Faulk, M. (1985) Secure facilities in local psychiatric hospitals, in *Secure Provision* (ed.) L. Gostin, Tavistock Publications, London, pp. 69–83.

Gostin, L. (ed.) (1985) *Secure Provision*, Tavistock Publications, London.

Gunn, J. (1985) Psychiatry and the Prison Medical Service, in *Secure Provision* (ed.) L. Gostin, Tavistock Publications, London, pp. 126–52.

Gunn, J., Maden, A., and Swinton, M. (1991) *Mentally Disordered Prisoners*, Report to the Home Office, HMSO, London.

Home Office (1990) *Provision for Mentally Disordered Offenders*, Home Office Circular No. 66/90, London.

Home Office and Department of Health and Social Security (1974) *Interim Report of the Committee on Mentally Abnormal Offenders*, Cmnd 5698, HMSO, London.

Home Office and Department of Health and Social Security (1975) *Report of the Committee on Mentally Abnormal Offenders*, Cmnd 6244 (The Butler Report), HMSO, London.

Lewis, P. (1980) *Psychiatric Probation Orders: Roles and Expectations of Probation Officers and Psychiatrists*, Institute of Criminology, University of Cambridge, Cambridge.

NACRO (1993) *Community Care and Mentally Disturbed Offenders* Policy paper 1, NACRO, London.

NHS Management Executive (1994) *Introduction of Supervision Registers for Mentally Ill People from 1st April 1994*, Health Service Guidelines HSG (94) 5, London.

Onyett, S. (1992) *Case Management in Mental Health*, Chapman & Hall, London.

Parker, E. (1985) The development of secure provision, in *Secure Provision* (ed.) L. Gostin, Tavistock Publications, London, pp. 15–65.

Royal College of Psychiatrists (1993) *Community Supervision Orders*, A Report of the Royal College of Psychiatrists, London.

Special Hospitals Service Authority (1991) *Within Maximum Security Hospitals: A Survey of Need*, SHSA, London. (Unpublished)

Walker, N. (1985) *Sentence Theory Law and Practice*, Butterworths, London.
Williams, J. (1990) *The Law of Mental Health*, Fourmat Publishing, London.

FURTHER READING

Home Office (1991) *Police and Criminal Evidence Act 1984 (S. 66) Codes of Practice*, revised edn., HMSO, London.

3

Inequality, discrimination and the mentally disordered offender

The aim of this chapter is to clarify the nature of discrimination towards mentally disordered offenders, to review the evidence that exists about inequalities and discrimination and to suggest ways in which this understanding can inform the practitioner in the field. The topics of discrimination, inequality and prejudice are all large ones and each could occupy a chapter in its own right. The intention is to avoid the 'paralysis of analysis' and to make discussion as succinct as possible with the guiding principle being relevance to practice. Not all inequalities arise from unfair discrimination and even if they did it is doubtful whether mental health workers have a great deal of power to change such inequalities. Nevertheless, it is important that professional judgements and practices do not reinforce or amplify inequalities and discrimination that can be found in wider society. To this end, this chapter highlights how this can occur and seeks to raise the consciousness of those who may not have thought that there was any cause for them to review their practice. The first aim is to eliminate unfair discrimination; the second is to encourage positive moves that help reduce inequalities and counteract the effects of discrimination. The topics covered will be discrimination against mentally disordered offenders as a group, racial discrimination and sex discrimination. These as a group, racial discrimination and sex discrimination. These will all be treated separately since each raises different practice issues. In reality these dimensions of discrimination may overlap and coexist but it is difficult to do justice to such complexities other than on a case-by-case basis.

WHAT IS DISCRIMINATION?

Inequality is an escapable part of the human condition. It exists in relation to wealth, intelligence and beauty to name but a few. Though some political philosophies such as socialism incorporate equality in relation to wealth as an objective, for the most part this is not seen as an appropriate goal or principle for professional practice. However, equality of opportunity commands widespread support particularly in relation to the public provision of services such as education and health, and this is also true in relation to employment in both the public and the private sector.

Prejudice also seems to be an inescapable part of the human condition and it is common to find actual differences between groups reinforced by myths and stereotypes. This is a feature of identifying with a group and goes with a sense of an in-group and an out-group, or 'us and them'. There is no law against being prejudiced for the simple reason that it would be impossible to enforce. However, if prejudice is translated into discrimination – treating individuals or groups differently – and that discrimination is not based on relevant criteria, then unfair discrimination is taking place. If this discrimination is on the basis of gender or race, it is illegal. If it is on the basis of mental illness, it may not be illegal but it is certainly not compatible with professional codes of conduct.

Campbell and Heginbotham (1991) give the example of a man whose treatment for renal failure was discontinued because his mental illness was considered by the responsible doctor to be preventing him from benefiting from treatment and was disrupting the treatment of others. It would appear that the doctor was operating on the basis of there being more deserving cases and if this was so then clearly that was unfair discrimination. However, if the sole reason had been the disruption of the treatment of others then it would be arguable that that was a relevant criterion, though one would still need to be convinced that all difficult and disruptive patients were being treated in this way and not just those suffering from mental illness.

Though discrimination may be openly expressed, it is more often disguised or covert. This may be because the person who is discriminating unfairly is aware of this but does not wish to be seen to be doing so, such as when 'No Vacancies' actually means 'No Vacancies for the likes of you' (mentally disordered, black, Irish or whatever). Discrimination may also appear in an unconscious or unthinking way without the person involved being aware of behaving badly or being unfair. This happens when discrimination is culturally supported and much sex discrimination falls into this category. Barnes and Maple (1992) present research findings that support the assertion that the criteria used for assessing mental health commonly involve different criteria being used for men and for women. This is not the only factor that needs to be considered in explaining why women have a higher rate of admission to psychiatric hospitals and units, but it is an important one.

A further aspect of this topic is indirect discrimination. This occurs when the general application of a rule or condition has a differential impact on one group rather than another. It also has to be shown that the rule or condition is not a relevant one. In the Reed Report (1992) (D of H/HO) an example of this is provided in relation to admission criteria for hostels. The criterion is that the potential resident should not be abusing drugs or alcohol. The application of this rule has a differential effect on mentally disordered offenders as that group has a higher than average rate of drug and alcohol abuse. As a result they are more likely to be turned down for a place. However, some thought would need to be given to the question of whether abuse of drugs or alcohol is a relevant criterion or not. Many would argue that it is and that the answer to the problem identified in the Reed Report is to have more hostels catering for mentally disordered offenders (which would accept those who had a history of drug or alcohol abuse) rather than expecting all hostels to accept such referrals. A further case study may provide a clearer example.

Case study

> A probation hostel which admits mentally disordered offenders has a requirement that all residents who are not in work must take part in the daily programme. The only exception to this general rule is where physical illness confines a person to bed. Mental illness is not accepted as a basis for non-participation. When a resident who suffers from depression is repeatedly unable to get up in time for the daily programme, breach proceedings are brought.

In this case a general rule is being applied but it is likely to impact more on those suffering from depression than other residents. Furthermore, it is hard to argue that ability to get up in the morning is a relevant criterion if it can be waived for those who are physically ill. This does not mean that failure to get up should be ignored for if it continued long-term the resident would not be obtaining the benefit of taking part in the daily programme. The answer is to view the behaviour as symptomatic of depression rather than as failure to comply with the rules of the hostel. However, the hostel warden might well defend the rule by saying that all residents are treated the same and therefore there is no unfair discrimination. A good understanding of indirect discrimination is important in such situations.

DIFFERENT FORMS OF DISCRIMINATION

The first form of discrimination to be discussed is that against mentally disordered offenders as a group and this usefully highlights the contrasts between different forms of discrimination. The difference hinges on the fact that a mentally disordered offender does differ from the average citizen in two important respects: being mentally disordered and having committed offences. It is therefore quite reasonable for these facts to be taken into consideration by key decision-makers such as hostel wardens, prison officers, police sergeants, doctors, magistrates, social workers and psychiatric nurses. In fact, the discussion in Chapter One included the point that all these key people are asked to take this into consideration in deciding how best to deal with them – what might be called fair discrimination. The difficulties arise when unfair discrimination creeps in and prejudice rather than professional judgement becomes the basis for deciding what should be done with and for the mentally disordered offender. In such situations individuals may be assessed as far more dangerous than they actually are, or alternatively their symptoms of mental illness may be viewed as malingering and psychiatric treatment withheld or delayed.

Racial discrimination is very different from this because race should not be a consideration in making a psychiatric assessment or in estimating the dangerousness of an individual patient or offender. This means that the inclusion of information about racial origin in reports and notes is usually indicative of prejudice and discrimination slipping into professional judgement. However, there are situations where this would not be the case and it would be unsatisfactory if the reader assumed that a colour-blind approach was being proposed. For example, it would be important to challenge a proposal to put a single black prisoner into an all-white wing of a prison where racism was rife. In that situation, race or skin colour is a relevant criterion for an assessment not because it tells us anything about the character of the person but because of the social context of race relations within the prison.

The word black will be used in a political rather than a literal sense to describe all non-white groups. It is recognized that not all members of such groups accept such a label but the argument for doing so is that despite their differences they have a shared experience of being discriminated against on the basis of being non-white. This seems to be an acceptable reason for using such language in a book such as this where a general position has to be adopted. However, the practitioner can be more sensitive to the views and feelings of individual black clients and care needs to be taken in exploring any person's self-concept in terms of race and colour. It is not appropriate for the white practitioner to tell a client that he should think of himself as black!

A distinction also needs to be drawn between race and ethnicity: the former is defined essentially by external characteristics such as skin and eye colouring and hair type, and the latter by internal characteristics such as culture, religion, language and identity. Culturally distinctive clothing and hairstyles provide an exception to this basis for division but it remains true that ethnicity is usually something that we have a choice about going public on while this is not true for race. Any service that seeks to meet the basic human needs of its clients should pay attention to these internal characteristics if it is to be accepted and used. Ethnic sensitivity is therefore an essential consideration in planning and delivering mental health services. This is why it is perfectly acceptable for a residential centre to develop its services on the basis of a distinctive ethnic or religious ethos. It is a different matter to do this on the basis of race and certainly a 'Whites Only' hostel would not be lawful or acceptable. However, there are examples of hostels which have all black staff as a matter of policy and most referrals are of black people. The rationale for this is the pervasiveness of racism in society and the need to create a safe haven from racism for black people. It is argued that race is therefore a relevant criterion in this context. Fernando's analysis of racism as a cause of depression provides strong support for such a position (Fernando, 1991).

Sex discrimination raises different issues from race although the legislative framework is similar. Clearly there are biological differences between men and women and there are situations where these are relevant as criteria for treating men and women differently. However, these tend to be overstated and as a result unfair discrimination does occur. For example, recruitment to the professions has historically been dominated by men. This is changing fast and some medical schools now have more female than male undergraduates. This suggests that there was no fair justification for the previous pattern of recruitment and that both direct and indirect discrimination were involved.

A further major difference between sex and racial discrimination is that women are far from a minority group and in fact are slightly in the majority in the UK. This means that gender issues are part of everyone's life with mixed gender households being the experience of the majority of people. So whereas some white people can distance themselves from issues of racism because they do not have a personal relationship with

a black person, this is untenable in relation to sexism.
Discrimination, inequality and prejudice related to gender are
thus part and parcel of both the personal and the professional
in the caring professions. Inevitably this means that there is
always a danger of personal views on what is appropriate
behaviour for a man or a woman spilling over into professional
assessments of the personal and social functioning of male and
female patients and offenders.

THE POWER OF THE WORKER

What all these forms of discrimination have in common is that
some groups in society are on balance likely to be disadvantaged compared to others. The detailed discussion of the
possible processes of discrimination will indicate which of these
are within the control and influence of the caring professions
and which are not. Emphasis will be given to those that are
within the professional ambit and this means that workers need
to accept they have power. They also need to accept that such
power can be exercised fairly or unfairly and that cumulatively
these individual decisions lead to groups of people receiving
or not receiving social justice.

Many people reading this book may not feel particularly
powerful and it may be helpful to clarify what is meant by
power. Those in the frontline of community care are usually
at practitioner level and are unlikely to feel powerful in relation to their own organizaiton. This will be particularly true
for those in training who have student status and may well
be placed in a team or unit on a short-term basis. Nevertheless,
the reality is that even the lowliest member of staff has a great
deal of power in relation to clients and residents. This can be
analysed in terms of statutory powers and these are indeed
a reality when dealing with mentally disordered offenders who
are often familiar with compulsory 'admissions' to psychiatric
and penal institutions. However, the most profound source
of power that staff members hold over clients and patients is
the power to define the situation. If there is more than one
view of a situation, a piece of behaviour or a person's suitability for an activity, the view that will usually hold sway is
that of the member of staff. An everyday example of this is
provided by the varied responses that might be made to a

hostel resident asking for assistance with a social security matter. Without knowing the person and their history it would be difficult to decide whether or not it was appropriate to offer help but it would be easy to make the decision purely on the basis of the worker's feelings towards the resident or of the worker's inclination to make a telephone call. Decisions like these are small change in the currency of power and yet it is through these minor matters that residents become aware of those staff who exercise power in a responsible and thoughtful way and those who do so in an arbitrary and unfair way. Either way power is being exercised and all workers need to come to terms with the implications of that for themselves.

There are significant differences between the power of the worker in field and residential work. In a residential setting the territory is the worker's and the worker is supported by a team and an ethos, a hierarchy and an agreed set of rules which others will enforce if one staff member fails to do so. It is also true that most residential settings are in some sense home, however temporary, to residents. This means that the group and the setting provide the primary context for the resident's life. This potentially puts staff in a strong position for they have available two potent sanctions: exclusion from the group and expulsion from the unit. In the latter the resident is rendered homeless and in the former he loses the support of the group. The more dependent the resident, the greater the power of both these sanctions.

Where staff have little or no power to expel, for example in prisons and special hospitals, power may be exercised in more brutal and physical ways, and sadly this is something that has to be faced though not accepted in this field of work. In less secure settings such brutality seems to be less common, presumably because there are more opportunities for the public to become aware of what is going on but also because staff retain the ability to expel and reject. In institutions of last resort this power is not available and staff and 'residents' are stuck with each other, sometimes with disastrous consequences. The Institute of Race Relations (1991) report entitled *Deadly Silence – Black Deaths in Custody* provides frightening reminders of this with examples of deaths in police custody, prison and secure hospital accommodation.

For those engaged in fieldwork the situation is and feels very different. When visiting a client in his home, many of the sanctions for residents and supports for the worker are absent. In addition the normal conventions are that the host rather than the visitor makes the rules in a person's home. This can leave the worker feeling powerless and may inhibit him from making the necessarily intrusive demands of, for example, a social supervisor. However, it may be helpful to remember that the worker still carries the power to define the situation that was discussed earlier. Indeed, the lack of other staff and residents may mean that a worker has fewer checks on his use of power and the client has no-one else to appeal to for fair play. Some fieldworkers such as probation officers and approved social workers may also have a far clearer statutory role of which the client will be aware.

THE POWER OF THE CLIENT

The power of the client in relation to the worker is a fascinating one and it is an issue that is likely to loom large at the early stages of a professional career, or when staff are changing their professional setting from an institutional to a community-based one. Despite the points made in the previous section, many workers do feel that clients are powerful and understanding this feeling is an important issue. A useful insight into the nature of the problem can be gained from the field of family therapy with children who are perceived by their parents to be out of control. Very often this will be framed as a child not doing as he is told and an important part of assisting the parents is to try to help them see that this is an unreasonable expectation. Indeed, the pursuit of a goal of total obedience is highly likely to produce the opposite to what was intended and this is something that staff and parents can usefully reflect on. A second element in helping parents in such a situation is to acknowledge that it may feel as if the child has a lot of power but that this is essentially 'down-power': that is the power to make things worse, to spoil and to destroy. Parents on the other hand have 'up-power' and need to use this to take control of the situation, to let go of their sense of powerlessness and make plans that can improve the situation for the child and for themselves. Part of this will involve engaging the child in the solution of the problem and in particular taking some responsibility for their behaviour.

A similar analysis can be brought to bear in relation to work with mentally disordered offenders, and workers will have to come to terms with the fact that having statutory power over someone does not necessarily mean that they will do as they are asked or directed. Equally important, workers need to face that negative or 'down-power' can be destructive and dangerous and that they as well as the client have a responsibility for making plans to avoid situations where this is likely to develop. This point will be returned to in Chapter Four on assessing risk.

HOW DOES DISCRIMINATION HAPPEN?

Prejudice is thoughts and feelings, while discrimination is essentially about decisions and actions. To fully understand what discrimination feels like is difficult unless we have been on the receiving end of such discrimination. Nevertheless, it is possible for workers to understand the processes involved. To do so it is necessary to have sense of the systems in which both worker and client are a part. Goldberg and Huxley (1980) provide a clear picture of the mental health system in the accompanying table (3.1) which they call 'The filter system at work in psychiatry'. Their table shows the process that occurs in sifting those with mental health needs out of the general population and it indicates the characteristics of each of the four filters through which an individual would pass in order to be admitted to a psychiatric bed. The actual rates indicate how much influence the key individuals play in the process. The primary care physician can be seen to play by far the greatest role, being central to both the recognition of mental disorder and the decision to refer to a psychiatrist. Social workers and community psychiatric nurses play a pivotal role when the primary care physician and/or the psychiatrist is weighing up whether the patient can be managed in the community or whether admission to a psychiatric bed is required.

Similar processes occur in the criminal justice system and it is not difficult to see that for both systems most of the filtering takes place at the community levels: the general

Table 3.1 The filter system at work in psychiatry

	the community	primary medical care		specialist psychiatric services	
	Level 1	Level 2	Level 3	Level 4	Level 5
	Morbidity in random community samples	Total psychiatric morbidity, primary care	Conspicuous psychiatric morbidity	Total psychiatric patients	Psychiatric in-patients only
One-year period prevalence, median estimates	250	230	140	17	6 (per 1000 at risk per year)
Characteristics of the four filters	First filter illness behaviour	Second filter detection of disorder	Third filter referral to psychiatrists		Fourth filter admission to psychiatric beds
Key individual	the patient	primary care, physician	primary care physician		psychiatrist
Factors operating on key individual	severity and type of symptoms, psycho-social stress learned patterns of illness, behaviour	primary care interview techniques personality factors training and attitudes	confidence in own ability to manage, availability and quality of psychiatric services, attitudes towards psychiatrists		availability of beds availability of adequate community psychiatric services
Other factors	attitudes of relatives availability of medical services, ability to pay for treatment	presenting symptom pattern, socio-demographic characteristics of patient	symptom pattern of patient, attitudes of patient and family	symptom pattern of patient, attitudes of patient and family	symptom pattern of patient, risk to self or others, attitudes of patient and family, delay in social worker arriving

Reproduced with permission from Goldberg, D. and Huxley, P. (1980) *Mental Illness in the Community: the Pathway to Psychiatric Care*, Tavistock Publications, London.

practitioner and the police respectively. Nevertheless, the contribution of professionals such as community psychiatric nurses, social workers and probation officers should not be underestimated for they both contribute their share to this filtering and they are often well-placed to influence the decisions of others. The confidence of a general practitioner to cope with a mentally ill person will often relate directly to the perceived availability and competence of community psychiatric nurses and social workers.

What can the worker do about inequality and discrimination?

The preceding section made clear that the direct efforts of the workers for whom this book is written are unlikely to make a major effect on the statistics of inequality – but even a minor contribution is significant. The fact that we can only do a little should not become an excuse for doing nothing. To do nothing is not to remain neutral: 'If you're not part of the solution, you're part of the problem.'

Workers also need to take responsibility for influencing key personnel. This could be in the ways suggested in the last section but attention could also be given to policy issues such as the monitoring of equal opportunities polices. Often policies are developed but insufficient attention is given to the hard slog of implementation. Further suggestions about what the worker can do will be found in the following three sections where each form of discrimination will be discussed in terms of the facts, the explanations of the facts and the implications for the worker. These implications will be examined at the level of the worker's self, direct work with the mentally disordered offender and work with others on his or her behalf.

DISCRIMINATION AGAINST MENTALLY DISORDERED OFFENDERS

It is generally accepted that the public and indeed many professionals hold negative and stereotyped views of those with a mental disorder. The same could be said with equal validity about offenders and it is therefore fair to describe this client group as doubly stigmatized and disadvantaged. Much

of the evidence for this can be gleaned from personal experience of trying to obtian employment or accommodation for
such clients. It may also be evident in public meetings such
as those held to appeal or protest against planning permission being granted for mental health or probation hostels and
daycentres. Similarly, press and television coverage of court
cases about mentally disordered offenders can provide depress-
ing confirmation of the depth and nature of prejudice in
society. Such impressions do not provide reliable evidence
about the extent and range of views that are held by all
members of the public.

Sayce (1994) reports that a representative sample of 1000
adults interviewed in January 1994 revealed a surprisingly high
level of support for community care of those suffering with
mental disorder (72%). The survey, commissioned by MIND,
showed that 76% supported the idea of a legal right to a
24-hour-crisis service and 67% were prepared to accept a small
tax rise to fund community care policies. Fifty-four%, however,
were concerned about the risk to the public and sought government reassurance that persons who posed such a risk would
not be discharged into the community.

It would be helpful to know why some employers and
landlords are prepared to accept mentally disordered offenders
and others are not. In the absence of research evidence the
individual worker is left to rely entirely on professional judgement to assess the situation. For example, what might we make
of a raw piece of data such as the fact that a particular landlord
had a track record of offering accommodation to those discharged from psychiatric hospital? On the face of it, this would
appear to be evidence of positive discrimination towards a
stigmatized client group and there are indeed some landlords
who can be particularly helpful. However, if the mental health
worker looked into the situation it could well emerge that the
rooms on offer were dirty and small, in a rough part of town
and being let at high rents. This is not an unknown scenario
and it speaks more of exploitation of vulnerable people rather
than positive steps to counter injustice and unfair discrimination.

Despite this caveat about the lack of hard evidence, it is
reasonable to assume that mentally disordered offenders
suffer from a wide range of prejudice ranging from the 'Mad

Axeman' to the 'Village Idiot'. However, it is worth noting that one in every six people will suffer from mental illness during their lives (Campbell and Heginbotham, 1991). This means that most adults will have a friend or relative who has had that experience as part of their lives. This does not necessarily lead to less prejudice but it can do so. Anecdotal evidence suggests that such personal knowledge can make a critical difference, for instance in a police officer's ability to differentiate between an arrested person who is quiet and one who is depressed and suicidal.

Accepting that prejudice and discrimination are a fact of life both for the mentally disordered offender and for those who work with them, what should be the priorities for the worker? These can be conveniently divided into work on self, direct work with the mentally disordered offender and work with others.

Work on self

No professional can insulate himself from the values and attitudes that prevail in society. Professional people are citizens too and they are as likely as the next person to have fears about their houses being burgled, their children or themselves being attacked. Those who often work with offenders may have had the opportunity to work out their feelings about these matters and to resolve conflicts between their personal anxieties and their professional responsibilites. However, many mental health workers do not have this experience and they may need considerable help when moving into this field. Likely responses include over-anxiety, where the worker cannot see beyond the offence to the person in need, and denial, where the worker behaves as if the offence is simply a matter of record and need not be considered in the present. A balance between these two extremes is important, as is the opportunity to discuss any particular issues that may arise for a worker. A common example of this is a personal experience of being a victim of a similar offence in the past.

This sort of work can usefully go on in supervision though a great deal depends on the supervisor's ability to create a safe enough atmosphere in which such anxieties can be shared.

Alternatively, group supervision or a training event can be arranged when a number of workers are starting to work with offenders, for example, the whole staff group of a hostel which has decided to start accepting mentally disordered offenders. A simple but effective device is to use press-cuttings of a recent case involving a mentally disordered offender as a starting point for a discussion of reasonable and unreasonable fears.

Just as some workers will need help with becoming aware of their feelings and attitudes about offending, so others will need help in relation to mental disorder. This again is an area where fears and fantasies are widespread and ignorance about the nature of mental illness can be a real stumbling block. This can be true for experienced, trained staff such as probation officers (Hudson *et al.*, 1993) as well as for students and untrained staff working in hostels and daycentres. Supervision and group discussion are again important, as is the transmission of factual data. As a general rule, attitudes and values are best addressed in small groups while information-giving can take place in large groups, in written or in audio-visual form.

Most workers, whether experienced or not, will need help with reconciling their personal and professional attitudes about mentally disordered offenders as this area of work tends to raise both realistic and unrealistic concerns about such matters as how predictable people are, how legitimate it is to interfere in people's lives and about the exercise of power and control. Intuition and 'gut feelings' often play a large part in such considerations and it is important that as far as possible these important 'tools of the trade' are used in a fair, unprejudiced way. The education of one's intuition is returned to as a topic in Chapter Four under the assessment of risk.

Direct work with mentally disordered offenders

Prejudice and discrimination are likely to affect all aspects of living from housing and employment through to the use of leisure facilities and forming personal relationships. From the point of view of the mentally disordered offender, this adds up to the reality or the threat of rejection in every area of life. Some will fight this with anger, some will approach it with weary acceptance, others will see it as just punishment for their offences – and indeed all these responses may be found in one individual over a period of time. Whatever the response the effects can best be understood sociologically in terms of spoilt identity (Goffman, 1990) and psychologically in terms of a profound and negative impact on self-esteem. This then is the starting point for anyone seeking to establish a professional relationship with such a person. The worker should not be surprised if feelings of worthlessness and self-loathing, anger and despair appear as a major issue at any stage in their direct work.

Combating such internalized negative stereotypes is not easy, particularly if the nature of the person's offences and/or their behaviour makes reassurance and unconditional positive regard difficult if not impossible. However, building up self-esteem through small achievements is a realistic and important goal and should provide some positive experiences to balance the negatives or deficits that also have to be addressed.

Offering a service that is free from prejudice and discrimination is an important goal for any worker or team. The world outside, however, is not under the control of the worker and therefore preparing clients for this unfair world is of key importance. This is likely to find a focus in relation to tasks like helping the client to prepare for a job interview, or disclosing information about offending or being in psychiatric hospital to a new friend. Role-playing the scenarios and rehearsing replies to the dreaded questions (Hollin and Trower, 1986) is all part of the work of combating discrimination against mentally disordered offenders.

Work with others

The 'others' covered by this heading may include family members, potential employers and members of the health, welfare or criminal justice systems. Prejudice and discrimination may be found among all these groups and effective advocacy will usually involve addressing this by a mixture of education, a challenging of stereotypes and listening to anxieties and worries. Because prejudice is likely to coexist with realistic anxieties about mentally disordered offenders, it is important to listen first so that any well-founded concerns can be addressed. This should reduce anxiety and may well lead to a reduction in unfounded fears.

In working with others who appear to be prejudiced, it is common to feel the need to make the particular client real by disclosing personal details. This is a difficult process even when it has been anticipated and discussed beforehand with the client. Recurrent problems centre on how much to disclose and whether to disclose all of it at the start. In dealing with a fellow professional the situation is fairly clearcut as any attempt to withold information would be seen as unprofessional and rightly so (the problem of incomplete referrals to hostels and daycentres is discussed in Chapter Seven). However, in dealing with a potential employer or landlord it is easy to say too much in an attempt to counter the blinkered views being expressed. In such a situation it may be helpful to reframe the task from 'selling' the client to seeking to understand and tackle the prejudice and fears being expressed: to shift the focus from the client's needs to the employer's attitudes and fears.

RACIAL DISCRIMINATION AND THE MENTALLY DISORDERED OFFENDER

Black mentally disordered offenders are at risk of discrimination in both the mental health and criminal justice systems. Statistics from a variety of studies over the last 20 years were drawn together in a discussion paper on Services for People from Black and Ethnic Minority Groups (D of H/HO 1992) for the Reed Report and some of these are summarized here. They show that black people who come to the attention of psychiatric services are more likely to be:

- removed by the police to a place of safety under Section 136 of the Mental Health Act 1983;
- detained in hospital under Sections 2, 3 and 4 of the Act;
- diagnosed as suffering from schizophrenia or other forms of psychotic illness;
- detained in locked wards of psychiatric hospitals;
- given higher dosages of medication

They are also less likely than white people to:

- receive appropriate and acceptable diagnosis or treatment at an early stage;

- receive treatments such as psychotherapy or counselling.

In detail, here are some of the statistics that are quoted in the
same discussion paper in support of the claims made above:

- 16% of Section 136 requests for approved social workers
  involved non-white people (10% Afro-Caribbean) compared
  with 6.4% in the study population;
- the average referral rate per 100 000 population was 116.7;
  - the average referral rate per 100 000 of the Asian
    population was 54.3;
  - the average referral rate per 100 000 of the Afro-
    Caribbean population was 204 (Barnes and Maple
    1990);
- the detention rate for first generation male Afro-Caribbeans
  is five times as high as for whites and for second generation
  male Afro-Caribbeans it is nine times as high (Cope, 1989).

The situation in the criminal justice system is no better and
is reflected in the following statistics from the same discussion paper. 'Studies over the past decade have established that
black people are more likely to be apprehended by the police
on suspicion of committing a crime; charged with a criminal
offence rather than cautioned; less likely to receive bail; more
likely to receive a custodial service.' The statistics to support
these statements include: 'Almost one in twenty young men
are likely to be sentenced to custody before reaching the age
of twenty-one. The proportion of young black men is nearly
one in ten (NACRO, 1986). 'In a West Yorkshire study of
probation-officer recommendations for community service
these were accepted by the magistrates in the following
percentages: 57% of white offenders; 30% of Afro-Caribbean
offenders; 13% of Asian offenders (Voakes and Fowler 1989).

Statistics such as these confirm that the situation is bad but
discrepancies such as the variation in rates of referral and
disposal for the Asian and Afro-Caribbean populations suggest
that a more detailed analysis may be required in order to
explain the facts or suggest how the situation could be
improved. These figures confirm the feelings in black communities that they receive less good a service than does the
white population and this alone is a powerful reason for

supporting the ethnic monitoring of all services. Without facts, it is all too easy to dismiss accusations of racism and discrimination as over-reaction to isolated cases and to avoid the difficult task of facing a bad situation and seeing how it can be improved. However, the presentation of these findings as percentages or rates per thousand can create the impression of a problem of unmanageable proportions; as a result, practitioners may be inclined either to despair or to dismiss the figures as unreliable. Neither response is of much benefit to the clients, offenders and patients requiring a service.

A different response is possible if such research findings are examined in more detail. For example the Barnes and Maple (1992) research, quoted above, covered 42 social services departments and produced data in relation to about one-third of the population of England and Wales (about 16 million people). However, the data on ethnic minorities was based on those ten local authorities where the black population exceeded 10% and these had a combined population of just over three million people. The percentage of referrals for assessment under the 1983 Mental Health Act were 12.6 of those of Afro-Caribbean origin and 6.5 for those of Asian origin. However, there were wide variations between authorities from 2.7–28.9% for Afro-Caribbeans and from 3–13.4% for Asians. Clearly, some authorities were being more successful than others in providing alternatives to compulsory admissions and it is important not to lose sight of this.

The total numbers may yield more manageable targets than the percentages do. Staying with the Barnes study, the total number of men compulsorily admitted from the ten local authorities was 696, and of these 48 were Afro-Caribbean. This means about five admissions of Afro-Caribbean men in each local authority per year. If this figure was reduced by one or two per year, the overall effect on the statistics would be impressive. How might this be achieved? Some answers can be found within that same piece of research. It showed that community psychiatric nurses were more likely to be involved wth Afro-Caribbean patients than other groups and also that Afro-Caribbean and Asian clients were more likely than other groups to receive continuity of input from social workers. This suggests that both services are already making considerable efforts to prevent compulsory admissions of black people to psychiatric hospitals and units. However, there were massive differences between black and white clients in terms of residential and day services with only one recorded use of daycare and one of day hospital for black clients. Voluntary support was much more frequent for both Asian and Afro-Caribbean clients than for their white counterparts. There were also lower rates of support from general practitioners for black patients. This provides a clear focus for service developments which would be likely to prevent unnecessary admissions for black patients.

A final but significant detailed finding from this research emerges from the demographic characteristics of the Afro-Caribbean and Asian groups. They were found to be very different with 40% of the Afro-Caribbeans being under 25 years of age compared with 13% of the white group, and only 6.2% of the Afro-Caribbeans being married compared with 53.6% of the Asians. The picture that emerges is of the extreme vulnerability of young single Afro-Caribbean males. This is also the most vulnerable group in relation to the criminal justice system and there is therefore a powerful argument for the development of specialist services for this group. However, the numbers involved in any one area may not be sufficient to warrant such separate provision, nor may every client wish to use such a service when it is available. It is therefore important that mainstream provision is reviewed to see whether it is in fact (if not by intention) a service for white middle-aged people. Assuming that this is the case, considerable work will need to be undertaken to ensure that services are genuinely accessible to all. Further suggestions about this can be found in Chapter Seven on residential and daycare services.

Work on self

Many articles and books addressing the problem of racial inequality and prejudice use the concept of racism to explain the situation. There are some difficulties in using this concept largely because it is a term which is used loosely. For example, most white people reading this book probably do not see themselves as racist. They probably identify racism with racial attacks, racial abuse and the daubing of racist graffiti. They might well accept that there is evidence of racism in parts of the British prison and special hospital system and where possible would seek to challenge such behaviour. That notion of racism is close to the Nazi ideology of racial superiority that sustained and justified Hitler's policies for the mass extermination of the Jews, gypsies, the mentally ill and the mentally handicapped during the 1930s and 1940s. There is little doubt that such attitudes are still present in British society and the recent election of a British National Party candidate in a London borough suggests that this type of racism is still an issue. The recent reports on Ashworth and Broadmoor Hospitals also show that there is no basis for complacency with regard to how these issues impact on black mentally disordered offenders.

However, a more pervasive and culturally supported form of racism is also present in British society and it is likely that all white people will have internalized this to some degree. It derives from our recent colonial past and from the fact that in that system the white man (and it usually was a man) was on the top of the pile, his language and culture was usually imported and superimposed on the indigenous people. Furthermore, in many countries there was a class system based on colour, with those of African origin making up a working class, those of Asian origin a middle class and those of European origin the ruling class. In some ways, this left British culture carrying a sense of each race having its place and an accompanying idea that each race should know its place.

Such belief systems have changed with time but it was interesting to hear a black student recently report on the frequent use of the adjective 'over-confident' in prison-wing reports about young Afro-Caribbean men. She was not sure of the significance of this until the same word was used about herself. There was little doubt that this comment arose from a sense that somebody did not know their place. Another version of this type of racism can be observed in relation to apparently positive comments, for example, about the prowess of Afro-Caribbean athletes and musicians, which are stereotypical and also suggest that perhaps that is all that Afro-Caribbeans are good at.

The general point here is that it is easy for white workers to become defensive when it is suggested that black patients and clients are encountering racist attitudes from professional staff. If such comments are made directly it may be helpful for all concerned to clarify what type of racism is being discussed. It will commonly be found that it is the latter type that is of concern but white staff may well react as if they are being accused of the former. This sort of confusion is unlikely to help the cause of race relations or the particular client, offender or patient. However, if white workers can take on board the idea that they are unlikely to have escaped the cultural baggage derived from recent colonial experience then a useful starting point will have been made.

Direct work with black mentally disordered offenders

The major issue here is whether a white worker can help a black person in need. The answer is not straightforward. In all the helping professions the central tool of the trade is the relationship between worker and client and at the core of this is good communication and empathy. As Philip Rack (1982) points out this is most easily established when there is a shared culture and internal landscape. When there are differences of race and ethnicity the landscapes may be different and more time and effort is needed to establish understanding. There should be little surprise if it is difficult to establish rapport. The danger is that pressure of time may lead to this sort of communication problem being interpreted as an indicator that the client is unlikely to benefit from help that is relationship based, such as groupwork. This factor may well explain the overuse of medication and physical methods of treatment for black patients.

Concern about this type of issue and the sorts of research findings quoted has led some local authorities to consider what steps should be taken to address the needs of black clients. In 1985 Sandwell began such a process of policy review of their Approved Social Work services and when this was reported on in 1990 (Patel) it was clear that a central assumption had been the importance of race and ethnicity. There was a concern about over-representation of Afro-Caribbeans among those compulsorily admitted to hospital under the Mental Health Act. 'A policy was devised that no person should be subject to an ASW assessment without a worker from the same ethnic group being present to provide guidance on racial and cultural matters (Patel, 1990, p. 29). The recruitment of Afro-Caribbean ASWs became a priority, as did the secondment of existing Afro-Caribbean staff for ASW training. Rotas were set up of staff who were prepared to advise when white workers found themselves assessing black clients. The obvious danger of exploiting black staff was avoided in this situation by a stand-by payment for those willing to go on the rota. In its first 18 months of operation, the policy had achieved its objective and only two admissions had occurred without the presence of a member of the appropriate ethnic group. This shows that such a policy is possible in an area with a significant black population.

In areas with few black staff it is inevitable that white staff will be called on to provide a service to black clients and it is important that they accept this responsibility and challenge. However, it needs to be acknowledged that good will, commitment and cross-cultural training may not overcome all such barriers and that it may be appropriate to look elsewhere to meet the needs of black clients, particularly when statutory intervention is being considered. In fact the development of care management legitimizes such an approach. The care manager's task is to assess needs but the meeting of identified needs often occurs through purchasing services. For some clients this will mean buying in ethnically sensitive services, such as a psychiatric assessment by someone of the same ethnic background.

The use of interpreters is a crucial consideration in working with those for whom English is a second language or who have little understanding of English. It is important not to let the pressure of events excuse poor practice in this area. Relatives are still being used as interpreters. We do not have to adopt an entirely Laingian perspective to see the dangers of this in terms of making proper assessments of what is going on in a family and what can be done to help. Similarly, hospitals and other organizations still expect ethnic minority staff to act as interpreters. Rarely are they paid for this service (which exploits them) but this practice also carries major dangers arising from the incomplete translation of legal and medical terms and concepts. A professional interpreter is needed when important professional judgements are being made. An interpreter needs to be equally conversant with both languages and have a good grasp of the particular professional context. For example an approved social worker assessment involves a comprehensive exploration of alternatives to admission. If the interpreter becomes very affected by the family's feelings of desperation and anxiety, it may be difficult to carry out such an exploration sensitively.

Experience and trust between worker and interpreter is invaluable and can best develop through regularly working together. The worker's own skills in using an interpreter will also develop with experience. Important considerations are making questions and statement short and clear, avoiding double negatives and not being afraid to check things out when confusion develops. With time the slower pace of communication which interpreting requires can actually allow for more reflection on what is going on and can lead to better questions. The delayed effect also allows the worker to observe the impact of whatever is being translated. Inevitably, the worker has to rely on less information than would normally be available. However, it is possible that better use is made of this limited information and also that the very process is a useful counter to any inclination to jump to hasty conclusions. For fuller discussion of this important topic see Baker *et al.* (1991) and Shackman (1984).

A primary tool of all mental health professionals is the development of a personal relationship with the client and within this the importance of language and the capacity to empathize are central. It is therefore important to examine the possible impact of racial discrimination on both these and to become aware of how racism manifests itself in the use of language. The reader is asked to embark on an exploration of how everyday language carries the values of a culture. The history of Britain is very much a history of colonialism and now that many who have their origins in the former colonies are living in the United Kingdom the history from-the-top is being countered by a history-from-below. This is reflected in a challenge about the use of language and since the end of colonialism major changes have occurred in what is acceptable language. Nevertheless, there is still considerable resistance about this and the use of the word black to mean negative is still commonplace. It is hard for a white person to internalize what this means on an everyday basis but in its totality it amounts to holding 'black' as a negative reference point.

It is easy to see why a black person might have some reservations about identifying with a culture in which an important aspect of their identity is seen negatively. In relationship terms this is likely to be shown by a degree of reserve, suspicion or even hostility towards a white professional which is unsurprising but nevertheless difficult to respond to. Care with language and an awareness of black history go hand-in-hand in helping a worker to understand and work with feelings such as these.

Work with others

The black mentally disordered offender has the same needs as white members of this group for good advocacy and persistent resource finding. However, there are particular issues that relate specifically to black clients which may benefit from further exploration. For example, why is it that so few black people are using day services and hostels? The research cited earlier in this chapter that confirmed this also mentioned a higher-than-average reliance by black clients on community groups and the extended family. It would not be difficult to see how a white worker's belief that ethnic minorities look after their own might become a self-fulfilling prophecy, particularly if the black client was either not aware of the facilities available or perceived them as not being for him. The white worker therefore has to guard against slipping into this set of assumptions and be prepared to challenge them when they are articulated by others. It also needs to be accepted that some black clients will only be able to benefit from a setting that is geared to his cultural and racial needs. This can be seen as separatist and white workers may need to advocate strongly for the right to be different and for provision to be genuinely multicultural.

SEXUAL DISCRIMINATION AND THE MENTALLY DISORDERED OFFENDER

The facts about sexual inequalities in the psychiatric and criminal justice systems tend to pull in different directions.

Women are admitted to psychiatric hospital at a rate of 468 per 100 000 while the equivalent figure for men is 364 per 100 000 (figures for 1986 quoted in Barnes and Maple, 1992). Women are twice as likely to be taking tranquillizers and two-thirds of those taking anti-depressants are women (Barnes and Maple 1992). Women are also referred for assessments under the 1983 Mental Health Act at a higher rate than men. Barnes *et al.* (1990) found rates per 100 000 of 82.5 for women and 68.4 for men. Of those assessed, 52% of women and 50% of men were 'sectioned'. However, this apparent equalization of risk masks considerable gender differences with 'sectioned' men being significantly more likely to be single and under 35 years old and women more likely to be over 65 years.

Criminal statistics provide a rather different picture with 83% of offenders in 1989 being male, a statistic that had changed little in the preceding ten years. Another view of the same phenomenon is provided by the information that one-third of males will have a conviction for at least one offence by the age of 31, while this is true for only 7% of females. Looking further along the process of criminalization, the average number of female prisoners was 1770 out of a total of 48 600 in 1989. Women also fare better after leaving prison. Of those leaving prison in 1986, 42% of male adult offenders were reconvicted within two years whereas the equivalent figure for female offenders was 34%.

The fact that there are relatively few recognized female mentally disordered offenders does create problems of being a minority group. Devi (1992) in a chapter about caring for mothers and babies in secure settings reported that there were no provisions for female mentally disordered offenders to be admitted with their babies to medium-secure units. Devi also reported that 84% of women in regional secure units admitted under the 1983 Mental Health Act had a baby under the age of two years. Despite this, her survey of unit staff revealed a figure of 50% who were opposed to the development of such units.

The reasons for not admitting mothers with their babies to such settings were rehearsed and it appeared that they were similar to those advanced when mother and baby units were first opened in psychiatric hospitals in the 1950s and 1960s. These included fears for the baby's safety, either from the

mother or other patients, and concerns about the management
of children in a ward setting. In fact, no evidence of harm to
children was found and the reactions of many patients was
positive. Those who might have been irritated by the children
tended to avoid them. The presence of babies also made it
much more feasible to assess the mother-child relationship and
hence to make realistic plans for discharge.

The explanations

The over-representation of women in the mental health system
has been the subject of considerable debate within the feminist
movement. Much attention has been drawn to the psychiatriza-
tion of women's issues and the pathologizing of 'normal'
distress and unhappiness by labelling it as mental illness
(Barnes and Maple, 1992). Such an analysis focuses attention
on the criteria used for evaluating the social functioning of men
and women and draws attention to differences in expectations
according to gender. Such sex-role stereotyping seems a
particular problem in relation to the diagnosis of psychopathy
and Gorman (1992) points out that 60% of women in Ashworth
Special Hospital are there because of arson.

There are other types of explanations for the disadvantaged
position that women suffer within the mental health system.
The work of Brown and Harris (1978) does not focus on variations in diagnostic crieria to explain gender imbalances but
draws attention to aspects of women's lives which make them
vulnerable to forms of mental illness such as depression. The
fine detail of their research is important because it shows that
women are not *per se* likely to develop depression but that
women in certain situations are. The most vulnerable groupings are those who have three or more children under 14 living
at home, those who are not in paid employment, who have
lost their mothers in childhood or who lack an intimate,
confiding relationship. However, paid employment or an
intimate, confiding relationship could afford protection to those
who were otherwise vulnerable. Findings such as these are
consistent with social psychological explanations for depression with a key linking concept being the impact of life-events
on self-esteem and self-concept. Such an explanation offers
encouragement to all mental health workers to seek reasons

for depression and need to have some confidence that social and psychological changes can bring about change even in clinical depression.

However, with diagnoses such as schizophrenia there is far less reason to believe that purely social or psychological models will provide an adequate basis for intervention. Genetic and biological causes look to be far more central with this diagnosis and as a result there is less scope for discrimination as an explanation for any gender differences that may be found.

Work on self

For all psychiatric diagnoses there is some consideration of what is appropriate behaviour for a person of this age, sex and social background. This seems inevitable as any judgement about another's behaviour can only be made in a social context. The individual practitioner, however, needs to be aware that this judgement is based on a particular set of assumptions and to be sensitive to the fact. For female staff there is the challenge of bridging the gaps in assumptions and lifestyles that may arise from any differences of class, race, age and sexual orientation between themselves and patients and clients. Male staff also have those considerations to bear in mind as well as the difference in gender, which for female staff may be a bridge and a basis for empathy and acceptance. Men may overestimate their ability to make a relationship in these circumstances and some reflection on this can be profitable. Increasingly, male staff need to spend time together discussing what sort of work is appropriate for them to become involved in and what should be more appropriately left to female staff. Such a discussion could usefully include the degree of protection needed for staff as well as clients.

Work with female mentally disordered offenders

It is interesting to read that until 1967 male probation officers could not supervise female offenders (Parsloe, 1972). One wonders how such a radical proposal would be received in the 1990s! Yet it is clear that a percentage of female psychiatric patients have been abused by men and it is unlikely that they will find it easy to disclose or work on this with male staff. The implication is that all staff, but particularly males, need to become aware of the possible impact of their gender on both the therapeutic and the control aspects that are part and parcel of working with mentally disordered offenders.

By the same token, it is worth considering if there are male offenders whom female staff should not work with or should only do so in certain situations. The inquiry into the supervision of Daniel Mudd (Wiltshire County Council, 1988) revealed that though his social supervisor was a man, the hostel where he was placed was mixed and most of the staff were female. The indulgence he was shown by staff in relation to his treatment of female residents was worrying and it is arguable that he would have been better placed either in an all-male environment or at least with more male staff. Whether that would have saved the life of the female resident he eventually killed is impossible to say. What can be said more authoritatively is that any member of staff, male or female, should feel able to say that they are frightened by someone with whom they are working and to expect that fear to be listened to and acted upon.

Work with others

If gender issues are discussed by staff, then it is much easier to address the difficult situations outlined above. Such discussions can also open up fruitful ways of working with gender issues with clients. For example, an analysis of gender issues may result in some groups being closed to members of the opposite sex, whether as staff or clients. Alternatively, the challenge may be to model a male and a female member of staff working together in a co-operative and equal way.

More difficult situations arise when only some staff are interested and committed to examining gender issues and if these same staff are junior staff it is hard to bring about change quickly. Some conflict may be inevitable and alliances may have to be formed with colleagues from outside the team to bring about change and give support.

SUMMARY

This chapter has covered a great deal of ground about inequality and discrimination. Its aim was to raise the consciousness of professionals about those processes they might be part of or well-placed to challenge. Even if these lessons are learned and acted on, much inequality and discrimination will remain. Living with daily reminders of the injustices of society is one of the unacknowledged stresses of those in the caring professions. Somehow, each person has to find a way of finishing work each day and returning home to relative comfort, ease and security. The discontinuity between the lives of worker and client can be a source of real moral strain and personal unease. The discomfort this can induce has to be coped with and there is a danger of slipping into a belief system that somehow the disadvantaged have brought their troubles on themselves. Though there is likely to be some truth in this, it needs to be faced that such a belief is essentially a coping mechanism and that 'blaming the victim' is not a productive way forward. An alternative way of coping is for the worker to identify strongly with the underdog and to become the champion of the disadvantaged. A preparedness to be an advocate for the client is part of tackling discrimination and disadvantage. However, the worker should beware the danger of accepting too much guilt and responsibility for the injustices of society. It is painful enough working at the interface between society and vulnerable people without accepting total responsibility on behalf of both society and the mentally disordered offender.

REFERENCES

Baker, P., Hussain, Z. and Saunders, J. (1991) *Interpreters in public service*, Venture Press, Birmingham.

Barnes, M., Bowl, R. and Fisher, M. (1990) *Sectioned: Social Services and the 1983 Mental Health Act*, Routledge, London.

Barnes, M. and Maple, N. (1992) *Women and Mental Health: Challenging the stereotypes*, Venture Press, Birmingham.

Blom-Cooper, L. (1992) *Report of the Committee of Inquiry into Complaints about Ashworth Hospital*, HMSO, London.

Brown, G.W. and Harris, T. (1978) *Social Origins of Depression: a Study of Psychiatric disorder in Women*, Tavistock, London.

Campbell, T.D. and Heginbotham, C. (1991) *Mental Illness: Prejudice, Discrimination and the Law*, Dartmouth, Aldershot.

Cope, R. (1989) The compulsory detention of Afro-Caribbeans under the Mental Health Act. *New Community*, **15**(3), 343–56.

Department of Health and Home Office (1992) (The Reed Report) *Review of Health and Social Services for Mentally Disordered Offenders and Others Requiring Similar Services*, Final summary report, Cmnd 2088, HMSO, London.

Department of Health and Home Office (1992) *Services for People from Black and Ethnic Minority Groups*. A discussion paper, HMSO, London.

Devi, S. (1992) Caring for mother and babies in secure settings, P. Harrison and P. Burnard (eds) in *Aspects of Forensic Psychiatric Nursing*, Avebury, Aldershot.

Fernando, S. (1991) *Mental Health, Race and Culture*, Macmillan/MIND, London.

Goldberg, D. and Huxley, P. (1980) *Mental illness in the community*, Tavistock, London.

Goffman, E. (1990) Stigma: Notes on the Management of Spoiled Identity, Penguin, London.

Gorman, J. (1992) *Stress on Women: Out of the Shadows*, MIND, London.

Hollin, R. and Trower, P. (eds) (1986) *Handbook of Social Skills Training*, Pergamon, Oxford.

Hudson, B.L., Cullen, R. and Roberts, C. (1993) *Training for work with mentally disordered offenders. Report of a study of the training needs of probation officers and social workers*. CCETSW, London.

Institute of Race Relations (1991) *Deadly Silence: Black Deaths in Custody*, Institute of Race Relations, London.

NACRO (1986) *Black People and the Criminal Justice System: Summary of the Report of the NACRO Race Issue Advisory Committee*, NACRO, London.

Parsloe, P. (1972) Cross-sex supervision in the probation and after-care service. *British Journal of Criminology*, **12**, 269–79.

Patel, H.J. (1990) *A report on aspects of the ASW services in the Metropolitan Borough of Sandwell*, available from the Metropolitan Borough of Sandwell.

Rack, P. (1982) *Race, Culture and Mental Disorder*, Tavistock/Routledge, London.

Sayce, L. (1994) Power to the people. *Community Care*, 10.3.94, 14–15.

Shackman, J. (1984) *The Right to be Understood: a Handbook on Working with, Employing and Training Community Interpreters*, National Extension College, Cambridge.

Wiltshire County Council (1988) *Report of a Departmental Inquiry into the Discharge of Responsibilities by the Wiltshire Social Services Department in Relation to Daniel Mudd from his Release from Broadmoor in May 1983 until his Arrest in December 1986 for the Murder of Ruth Perrett*, Wiltshire County Council, Salisbury.

Voakes, R. and Fowler, O. (1989) *Sentencing, Race and Social Enquiry Reports*, West Yorkshire Probation Service.

4

The assessment of risk

THE HUMAN VOLCANO

When we consider issues of risk and dangerousness it is natural to think of settings where people who have demonstrated acts of violence are kept, such as special hospitals, secure units, prisons, etc. Indeed, there is often some kudos attached to those who work directly with people at the extreme end of the violence/risk spectrum. By working on a daily basis with offenders and/or patients who have acted out their aggressive tendencies, staff develop skills in managing such people in an institutional setting. Most importantly they work as a team, backed up by elaborate security systems and techniques for minimizing and controlling violent behaviour. Moreover, as staff spend many hours each day with those in their care, they quickly become familiar with an individual's changes of mood and demeanour. Staff are often aware, for example, of the possibility of difficulties from a patient on a particular day, by his demeanour on waking. The opportunities for such intimate contact enable staff to gauge the propensity for violent behaviour fairly accurately although there is always the possibility of the unexpected 'flare-up'. Even in these instances the staff team is able to fall back on well-rehearsed routines of intervention and containment.

By contrast, workers in the community are far more exposed to risk with considerably less support. Their clients are much more likely to be 'unknown quantities' in terms of risk potential. Opportunities to get close to the client in order to pick up early signs of difficulties are often limited to brief contacts which at best are likely to be only once or twice a week. Knowledge of the client's background may be scanty, particularly for those clients who have not been 'through the system'. Furthermore, many mentally disordered offenders in the community are notoriously difficult to keep track of, frequently moving from one lodging house to another, shunning regular attendance at daycentres and not always keeping appointments with supervisors or out-patient clients. Where some kind of statutory supervision is in place, there is recourse to some sanction for non-compliance but in many instances this will not be the case and the worker may not feel totally in control. There will be those clients who readily agree to supervision and support on a voluntary basis in order to avoid prosecution or receiving a custodial sentence, but who may be less than enthusiastic about subsequently receiving help.

Such reluctance is perhaps understandable when we consider that in most caring relationships the worker is likely to restrict the freedom and independence of the client. This is particularly so in relation to the mentally disordered offender where the worker is acting as an agent of social control. The worker has a responsibility not only to the client but also to the wider community and it may be difficult to reconcile the two. This is highlighted further when the worker is undertaking some form of compulsory supervision under relevant legislation. At times the worker may be seen as a threatening figure in view of his status and authority or perceived authority. In certain circumstances the worker will have actual authority to return an offender to court, to remove a person to hospital against his will or to take children into care. It is therefore not unusual for the worker to become a target for the client's hostile feelings.

Many clients will try to find a way of making good use of the support on offer without sacrificing too much personal control. In such situations Breakwell (1989) claims that violence against practitioners is hardly surprising. She takes the view that the client faces a double dose of distress: the original problem that caused the worker to be involved and the threat to self-determination that the worker comes to symbolize. The result is that clients who lack the ability to respond to such threats by sophisticated argument are likely to resort to violence. In this context, violence is a way of redressing the imbalance of power. This may apply particularly to the persistent anti-social offender who has a personality disorder rather than a formal mental illness and whose problems may be compounded by excessive long-term use of alcohol. Such clients are often unable to tolerate the constraints imposed upon them and resort to habitual aggressive behaviour as a way of asserting their independence.

In other cases, where the client suffers from a serious mental illness, violent behaviour may occasionally occur during an acute psychotic episode with either a marked delusioned state and/or loss of contact with reality. Such a condition is often associated with unbearable levels of internal tension. If the worker happens to be caught up in the client's delusional system, he may fall victim to unprovoked aggression as illustrated by the following example:

Case study

> Maurice had suffered from a chronic schizophrenic illness for a number of years and was sustained in the community by regular supervision from a community psychiatric nurse who also regularly administered a depot injection. The CPN had known Maurice for more than 18 months and had always found him to be placid and compliant. However, on one particular occasion when the nurse called at Maurice's home, he found him to be agitated and suspicious. As they walked together into the living room, Maurice suddenly turned and punched the nurse squarely in the face, breaking his nose. When seen by a psychiatrist later that day, Maurice said that the nurse was going to inject him with radioactive liquid.

Fortunately not all forms of violence result in death or serious injury, nor is it a normal day-to-day experience. Nevertheless, exposure to threats, minor assaults and risky situations are not all uncommon and are grossly under-reported (Rowett, 1986; Brown *et al.*, 1986). By the very nature of work with emotionally damaged and vulnerable members of society there will be occasions when the helping professional encounters the aggressive client. While there may be situations as described above when a worker may fall victim to an impulsive, quick and unprovoked attack, it is more usual for an incident to evolve from a sequence of events like frustration, effects of alcohol and the worker's mishandling of the situation. It is important therefore that the worker has some understanding of the likely components of personal characteristics and situational factors which may precede aggressive and/or violent behaviour.

As an analogy for the expression of violence in human beings it is useful to consider the features of a volcano which neatly illustrates the process involved. The reader will be familiar with the cone shape of a volcano containing a mixture of steam, gas and lava. The mixture is held in check by the chimney of the volcano being blocked by a plug of solidified lava from an earlier eruption. The onset of an eruption is marked by an increase in hot air and gases escaping from cracks and fissures in the mouth of the cone, together with a trembling of the earth and faint underground rumblings. A deafening explosion follows when the plug or crust of lava is blown out of the crater under the enormous pressure built up by steam and gas. People in the immediate vicinity may be injured or even killed.

When considering the human volcano we can see that the volatile mixture is made up by the interaction of personality and situational factors. Where environmental stress or threat exceeds the individual's capacity to cope comfortably, a violent potential is created. Fortunately, the human volcano also has a plug that stops it erupting every time anger is provoked. This plug is provided by inhibition or adherence to social conventions. However, the inhibitional plug tends to dissolve in alcohol and as a result of drug abuse. When this occurs, hot air starts to come out of the mouth of the human volcano in the form of invective and abuse until the inhibitional plug is breached and a violent eruption ensues. People in the immediate vicinity may be injured or even killed. This model is represented in Figure 4.1.

Just as there are many types of volcano, there are many different types of human volcano. And just as real volcanoes are not necessarily permanently of one type or another and may change their nature, the same applies with the human variety.

Most people tend to represent the dormant volcano. Everyone has a potential for violence but it is usually well beneath the surface and does not seek expression. An efficient inhibitional plug keeps feelings of tension under control and provides a large capacity to absorb a fair amount of

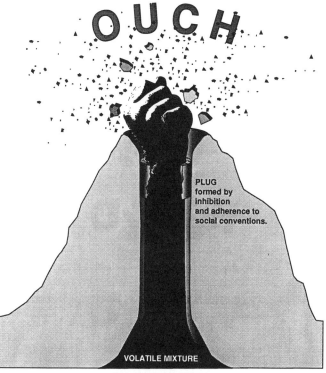

PLUG formed by inhibition and adherence to social conventions.

VOLATILE MIXTURE

formed by the interaction of
situational factors
(environmental stress and frustrations,
subculture where violence accepted, availability
of weapons, behaviour of victim, etc.) and
personality factors
(personality defects, presence of mental disorder,
low threshold to stress, etc.)
Plus effects of alcohol and drug abuse.

Figure 4.1 The human volcano

environmental frustration without resorting to violence. When anger is aroused, aggressive feelings are sublimated and/or displaced and are realeased in a socially acceptable way.

Nevertheless, there are those with over-controlled person-alities who act like an extinct volcano and who erupt suddenly and unexpectedly, often with devastating results. Such people have a strong inhibitional plug and adhere strongly to social convention. They tend to be compliant, are often even timid, unassertive and easily taken advantage of. As such, they find it impossible to express anger and their aggressive feelings are severely repressed. The result is a compression of all the anxiety and bad feelings into a small space, thus creating a great deal of pressure within. Because all the cracks and fissures in the inhibitional plug have been sealed up tight, there is no way of letting off steam. Outwardly, such people always seem calm and their violent potential is easily viewed as extinct. However, in exceptional circumstances when provocation is extreme or if the strong inhibitional plug is weakened by a depressive psychosis, the resulting explosion of violence can be tremendous with the effect that the victim of the violence is severely injured or even killed. Offenders who commit serious violence in the context of a psychotic depression often target their own families to relieve them of the trials of such a wicked world and follow their murderous act with a suicide bid. After the event, friends and acquaintances will often be heard to say how surprised they were at this behaviour, that it was totally out of character in a normally gentle, inoffensive person.

By contrast there are those who are always troublesome and who could be described as active human volcanoes. Just as normal active volcanoes are associated with faults in the earth's surface, the active human volcano is associated wth faults in a person's personality. The sort of person who falls into this category are those with under-developed and damaged personalities, those described as immature, sociopathic or psychopathic. Because of their shortcomings, their potential for violence is much greater than normal and their capacity to absorb environmental stress is greatly reduced. Their inhibitional plug is generally weak, particularly if they live in a subculture where violence is socially acceptable. The plug is also often permanently soggy through being soaked in alcohol or from the effects of drugs. The use of violence therefore is often considered an acceptable way of resolving difficulties by their peer group. If in the past this has met with success then the habit becomes reinforced and strengthened. The only consolation with this group is that violence tends to feed on the energy of youth, so that age mellows even the most habitual offender.

The other group that may be considered to be active human volcanoes are a small proportion of people with mental disorders. Although most forms of mental illness are characterized by fear, anxiety and lack of confidence rather than over-aggressive behaviour, there is a small proportion of sufferers who can be dangerous in a psychotic stage of their illness. Occasionally, the grossly paranoid and deluded patient may take up arms to defend himself against an imagined persecutor, or develop irrational beliefs about someone normally held dear. A local newspaper report records such an incident:

> schizophrenic . . . strangled and battered his 76-year-old grandmother to death after being invited to breakfast a court heard last week . . . He told people he decided to take her to sleep with him . . . and then he tried to smother her with a pillow before strangling her with a chain and hitting her several times with a glass vase.

Such offenders are likely to attract a hospital order and secure detention and subsequently need close supervision in the community. Great care needs to be taken to ensure that such an event does not reoccur and that risks are minimized in the future. For the professional working with the mentally disordered offender, the issues are complex. Not only is it necessary to minimize the risk to others but the worker must also take account of his own safety and the client's risk to himself.

RISK TO OTHERS

Assessing the risk of violent or dangerous behaviour is an imprecise art. There are no foolproof methods of predicting future behaviour, violent or otherwise. Nevertheless, professional judgements have to be made, from time to time, about the degree of risk that can be tolerated in any given situation and about the action needed to contain it. Probably the best way of anticipating future conduct is to gain an understanding of a person's previous behaviour patterns and, where violent incidents have previously occurred, to have detailed knowledge of the circumstances surrounding them. Where, for instance, a violent offence has been perpetrated, it is not enough simply to know the legal charge. Prins (1986) uses the example of rape to illustrate the point. He argues that 'there is an important qualitative difference between what might be described as "ordinary" rape and the type of attack where the offender ties the victim up, rapes her, renders her unconscious, brings her round again and then commits further assaults and so on.' The legal charge of rape gives no indication of the type of attack that occurred or any insight into the psychology of the attacker.

In many cases the relationship of the victim to the attacker is important. Some individuals are quite specific in their choice of victims and will not be violent to others. For example, spouse murders. It should be noted whether any particular individual is at risk, such as neighbours, a member of the family, an employer, etc., or whether a wider group is vulnerable such as minor boys at risk from the paedophile and adult women from the exhibitionist or rapist. Often the risk disappears with the immediate focus for aggressive feelings.

The importance of acquiring detailed information about previous violent incidents cannot be overstressed and as Scott (1977) says:

> it is patience, thoroughness and persistence in this process, rather than any diagnostic or interviewing brilliance that produces results. In this sense the telephone, the written request for past records and the checking of information against other informants, are the important diagnostic devices.

For those supervising 'restriction order' patients, much of the above work will already have been carried out and at the beginning of the supervision process the supervisor should have been thoroughly briefed and armed with the relevant information. Risk factors will have already been identified and catalogued. In other situations in the community, however, this may not be the case. Where the client has demonstrated being a risk to others in the past, it is crucial to undertake the necessray background investigation at the outset of contact or even before if possible.

It is perhaps reassuring that people are rarely spontaneously violent. Violent incidents are invariably the outcome of the interaction of personal and situational factors which can usually be identified. Prins (1986) argues that it is unhelpful to view the offence in isolation and more productive to identify its situational determinants. It is better therefore to think in terms of dangerous situations rather than dangerous persons. A helpful framework for assessing the total situation has been established by Scott (1977) in the form of the following equation: Offender + victim + circumstances = Offence.

Its application is demonstrated by the following example:

Case study

Brian, a 26-year-old man of limited intelligence and with a diagnosis of schizophrenia, was admitted to a regional secure unit under Section 37 of the Mental Health Act 1983, after attacking a woman in a public house. After eight months he was discharged by a Mental Health Review Tribunal to a supervised hostel. Voluntary supervision was offered by a community psychiatric nurse who also administered a depot injection on a fortnightly basis. Although there were copious notes on the case file, these had not been collated, nor had the offence been analysed in any detail. Using the above formula, the community psychiatric nurse was able to gain a much better understanding of the incident than was previously available:

Offender: in the weeks leading up to the offence Brian had become increasingly psychotic. Two months before he had stopped attending the GP surgery for his depot injection and nobody had followed this up. When not on medication he tended to develop paranoid delusions which appeared to be present at the time of the offence.

Circumstances: Brian had been living alone in a bedsit and had become rather isolated and lonely. He had recently lost his job as a storeman due to poor work performance. His loss and loneliness had led to feelings of depression and he had gone to the pub for a drink.

Victim: she was a young woman, unknown to Brian. However, she physically resembled Brian's younger sister who had teased him unmercifully in the past. She was with a group of friends at an adjoining table and was laughing a lot.

Offence: on hearing the nearby laughter, Brian thought it was at his expense. He had already drunk several pints of beer and on seeing the young woman laughing saw only his sister teasing him yet again. It was in this context that he moved across to her table and without any warning punched her in the face and set upon her with intent to strangle her.

With the above analysis the CPN was able to formulate a clear plan of action to reduce the risk of further incidents. It was important to ensure that Brian remained symptom-free and that his illness was strictly monitored. Any avoidance of medication by Brian would need to be vigorously pursued to avoid a re-emergence of his paranoid delusions. Rehabilitation plans would need to take account of Brian's difficulty in living alone and inability to socialize. Any subsequent loss in his life may require him to need additional support at that time. A brooding, paranoid Brian was to be avoided. As far as the victim is concerned it would be difficult to avoid Brian encountering young women but some account may need to be taken of the behaviour towards him of young female hostel staff or colleagues at work. They may need to be briefed on not appearing to be 'taking the mickey'. In Brian's case such measures should greatly reduce the propensity for violent behaviour in the future.

Where the client is known to have a propensity for violence, efforts must be made to ascertain the pattern of events that lead to each incident. In many instances, the display of aggressive behaviour may be much more generalized than the above example. Accordingly, when encountering a new client who may pose a threat to others, an extensive interview should be undertaken focusing particularly on the client's history. Questions should be frank and direct, as though one were questioning an individual who is suicidal. Monahan (1981) suggests that the following information about the client should be gathered by focused enquiry:

- how much has he thought about violence?
- what has he done about it?
- what weapons does he have?
- what preparations has he made?
- how close has he come to being violent?
- what is the most violent thing he has done?

A thorough probing of all forms of past violence should be conducted, paying particular attention to the recency, severity and frequency of violent acts. Whenever possible such information should be corroborated by a spouse, a relative or a friend. In subsequently assessing the probability of repeated violence the worker will need to consider:

- the characteristics that describe the situations in which the person reacts violently;
- the characteristics that describe the situations the person will confront in the future; and
- the similarity of the situation the person will confront in the future to those that have elicited violence in the past.

Armed with such knowledge it should be possible to limit the risk of further violence by reducing the individual's exposure to certain situations. Stenge (1977) also lists seven common precipitators to violence which, if avoided, will greatly reduce the propensity for such behaviour:

1. Much aggression is generated by fear, not only of physical threat but of loss of self-esteem and loss of freedom. It may also arise from the person's psychopathology, such as thinking that incorporates delusions of persecution.
2. A further feature of equal importance is frustration, particularly when arising from feelings of helplessness and where personal needs and desires are thwarted.
3. Anxiety about losing control may result in acting out behaviour to test out the worker's capacity to contain the situation. Thus some minor forms of hostile behaviour may occur to obtain assurance that the worker will provide support when necessary. The worker's response may determine future behaviour.
4. Unresolved conflicts arising from previous rejections, disappointments and hurts may cause anxiety, anger and guilt. Further failures may reinforce these feelings.
5. Feelings of inferiority may produce aggressive behaviour as a way of compensating for self-perceived shortcomings.
6. Intrusion of territory and personal space may also produce hostility.

7.　Anger as a component grief, if not dissipated, may lead to the carrying of negative feelings. Thus an individual who has lost a loved one, a job, their self-esteem or status must work through the grief process to avoid establishing a pattern of behaviour that could be considered disturbed.

Much of the abuse can be countered by the sensitivity of the worker to the client. At the outset of any new contact it is helpful to establish the ground rules of supervision or support. The client must understand the extent of the worker's authority while the worker should not be unnecessarily authoritarian. Above all, the worker will need to set clear limits but at the same time show respect for the client and avoid undermining his self-esteem. While an equal partnership may in reality be unattainable, it should be constantly strived for.

Occasionally, despite the efforts of the worker, clients may pose a risk to others either through a deterioration in their mental health or by being faced with provocation they cannot ignore. Some acutely violent people are afraid of their own violent urges and will seek help in controlling them. Bute (1979) talks of the importance of being firm and verbalizing the intention of helping the client keep control. Sometimes, talking through the person's violent feelings calmly and pointing out the consquences of further dangerous behaviour can be helpful. As Prins (1986) points out, such action may enhance the client's self-esteem and their feelings of being 'rational and in command'. Bringing things into the open may offer an opportunity of devising a coping strategy or simply diffuse the situation.

Where such measures do not work and a risk to others is still present, consideration must be given to some form of intervention. If the stressors that give rise to the client's aggressive response cannot be removed, then the client himself may need to be removed from the situation or removed from the community altogether. If, for instance, the client is attending a daycentre and starts threatening another attender, and their differences cannot be resolved, a temporary suspension may be necessary. Aternatively, a change to the pattern of attending could be adopted in order to avoid them being together on the same day. However, if the client's aggressive behaviour is due to a deterioration in mental health, medical intervention may be necessary including the use of hospital admission where appropriate. Ideally, clients should be encouraged to enter hospital on a voluntary basis but according to the degree of risk involved it may require the use of compulsory detention under the Mental Health Act 1983. 'Restricted' patients who have been conditionally discharged from hospital may be recalled by the Home Office if it is felt that the degree of risk is unacceptable. Others may need to be brought before the court to have any existing order modified or to be charged afresh for any new misdemeanours.

RISK TO THE WORKER

As with any other group of clients, work with the mentally disordered offender will expose the professional to a degree of risk. This forms a constant part of life for the professional helper and indeed the voluntary worker, although the former is more likely to arouse resentment and negative feelings by virtue of their control or perceived control over the client. This, together with the unsettled way of life of many clients who may also abuse alcohol and drugs, increases the vulnerability of the worker. A major study into violence in the health services conducted in 1986 by the Health and Safety Commission showed that one in 200 workers had suffered a major injury following a violent attack during the preceding year. A further one in ten needed first aid and one in 20 had been threatened (Health Services Advisory Committee, 1987). Similarly, a national survey of social services departments by Rowett (1986) showed an annual assault rate of one assault for 259 posts. Further analysis showed that 38% of the assailants of the subgroup studied had a history of one or more psychiatric admissions, 45% had been convicted of at least one criminal offence and 28% had convictions for violence. Perhaps even more interesting is the fact that 85% of assaults were committed by established clients whom the social worker had known for some time. Assaults by members of the client's family represented a further 10%.

Clearly, there is no room for complacency even when staff consider they have a good working relationship with the client. The fact that the client has not posed a threat in preceding interviews does not mean that he will not pose a threat at future meetings, particularly where there is a history of aggressive behaviour. The interaction between the two parties must be constantly reappraised. As well as considering possible triggers for aggressive behaviour in the volatile client, such as high levels of stress, misuse of drink or drugs, the development of paranoid delusions, etc., it is worth deliberating on one's candidacy as a potential victim. Breakwell (1989) has developed a useful 'dangerousness checklist' which should be applied to assess the risk of violence in a situation about to be entered into by the worker. The following questions the worker should ask himself have been extracted from the list as they seem particularly helpful in assessing whether violence is likely to be directed towards the worker:

- Has the person verbally abused me in the past?
- Has the person threatened me with violence in the past?
- Has the person attacked me in the past?
- Does the person perceive me as a threat to his/her children?
- Does the person think of me as a threat to his/her liberty?
- Does the person have unrealistic expectations of what I can do for him/her?
- Does the person perceive me as wilfully unhelpful?
- Have I felt anxious for my safety with this person before?
- Are other people present who will reward the person for violence?

In using the complete list the more questions that produce the answer 'yes', the greater the danger. Additional questions could be added to the list, such as:

- Have I become emeshed in the person's delusional system?
- Do I resemble in any way someone previously threatened or assaulted?

Where threats or actual violence have been an issue in the past, it is crucial that all those involved in the client's care are made aware of the situation. Workers standing in for colleagues who are on holiday or sick leave need to know whether there is a risk involved in seeing a client. Many agencies mark files, index cards and computer records of potentially violent clients in order to alert new workers to the possible risk. Mental health provider units are also required to maintain a register of any patient who is at risk of serious violence or suicide.

Similarly, cross-agency and cross-professional communication is vital in such cases. If a client is suffering from an active mental illness, it may require vigorous outreach activities to keep a reluctant customer in sight and within treatment. Failure to vigorously pursue the after-care of some psychotic ex-hospital patients have led to a number of recent tragedies. An inquiry into the tragic death of social worker Miss Isobel Schwarz who was killed by a former client, Miss Sharon Campbell, on 6 July 1984, revealed a failure of communication between the professionals involved and a failure to keep Miss Campbell in the system, to be contributory factors to the incident (DHSS, 1988). Similar failures of communication and liaison between agencies, lack of assertive outreach and the ignoring of warning signs and symptoms led to the tragic death of Jonathan Zito at the hands of Christopher Clunis, according to a later inquiry (Ritchie *et al.*, 1994).

Failure to communicate previous violence by a client exposed a new worker to attack in the following example:

Case study

Jennifer, an 18-year-old young woman accommodated by the local authority, was due for her six-monthly review. The reviewing officer (female) was new to the case and arranged the meeting in the staffed hostel where Jennifer was living. Two other members of staff were present. Immediately after the introductions were made and as they were about to sit down, Jennifer, without warning or provocation, hit the reviewing officer with a side swipe to the head. After the reviewing officer regained her composure, Jennifer remained agitated but calmed down after being given a cup of coffee. With everybody's agreement the review then proceeded. After a few minutes Jennifer suddenly threw her full coffee mug, hitting the reviewing officer on the head. Jennifer then tried to attack the reviewing officer but was restrained. The reviewing officer left the room, only to find that Jennifer quickly broke free and pursued her and attacked her once more. Fortunately, Jennifer was finally effectively restrained and no further damage was done.

The subsequent investigation into this case showed that Jennifer had attacked two previous reviewing officers (both female) during the course of a review. Although both attacks had been noted in the running records of the file, neither had been highlighted and there was nothing on the front of the file to indicate that these attacks had taken place. The reviewing officer had not had the full file before the review meeting and was unaware of the attacks to her predecessors. Furthermore, the senior member of staff present from the hostel thought that the reviewing officer did know and so did not bother to mention it. Jennifer had previously received psychiatric treatment and for several weeks before the review had become increasingly agitated. However, there had been some delay in getting her an out-patient appointment with her psychiatrist and this had not been pursued. It became clear that in Jennifer's mind female reviewing officers represented the despised authority of the agency and became the target for her pent-up feelings of anger and aggrievement.

Several lessons were learned from this incident:

1. Vital information about previous violent behaviour was not properly recorded. The records gave no indication of possible future risk, nor was any verbal information exchanged about the previous incidents. Not only was the reviewing officer unprepared to anticipate difficulties, but staff present who were aware of what had happened before made no allowances for this in the arrangements for the meeting.
2. Jennifer's deteriorating mental health had been left unchecked and attempts to arrange a mental health assessment had not been pursued vigorously enough.
3. The hostel staff and reviewing officer were foolhardy in allowing the review to continue after the first assault. To abandon the review at this stage would not be seen to be weak or shameful, just sensible. There is no point in trying to prove how brave one is and expose oneself to further abuse. Workers are not paid to take risks of this nature.
4. Once the violence had occurred, there did not seem to be any planned strategy for meeting it. Not only was there an *ad hoc* response but Jennifer was easily able to overcome the attempts to restrain her and make further attacks on the reviewing officer.

Good professional practice should not only ensure that risks are minimized as much as possible, but Section 7 of the Health and Safety at Work Act 1974 provides a duty of every employee to the employer to:

- take reasonable care for his own health and safety;
- take reasonable care for the health and safety of anyone who may be affected by his acts or omissions; and
- co-operate with his employer or any other person to enable legal obligations to be met.

There should be no occasion when a worker need go alone into a potentially dangerous situation or otherwise knowingly expose themselves to risk. Many employers now offer guidelines to staff for the prevention and management of violence by clients which are usually a combination of common sense and tried and trusted procedures. The following is a summary of some of the most common advice given to staff to minimize the risk of violence.

Anticipation/prevention

Emphasis should always be placed on predicting and preventing violent behaviour. As previously stated a thorough background knowledge of the client and potential trigger factors for violence is essential. Records of all clients with a known propensity for violent behaviour should be marked to alert new workers to the possible risks. Intervention strategies which have been found to be inflammatory should be highlighted. Where difficulties are anticipated the approach to the client should be carefully planned and adequate support be made available. In more specific situations, such as the admission of an actively resistant patient to hospital under a section of the Mental Health Act 1983, the occasion calls for considerable forethought and skill from the approved social worker to avoid the situation deteriorating into an undignified scuffle or worse (Vaughan, 1988). In short, before engaging with any client with a record of violent behaviour, workers should, as the well-known maxim states, 'be prepared'.

Home visiting

Where a risk of violence is evident, serious consideration should be given as to whether a home visit is really necessary.

Alternative arrangements such as an office-based interview are preferable in such circumstances. However, where a home visit is required, suitable precautions need to be taken such as visiting in pairs and/or seeking police assistance. In any event, steps should be taken to ensure that a responsible person knows where and when the visit is taking place so that assistance can be sent if the worker does not report back within a reasonble time. Some staff are also reassured by carrying a personal alarm.

Office settings

Reception facilities may well have a bearing on how a client reacts and should be designed to create a feeling of friendliness. Accordingly, they should be warm, clean and welcoming with up-to-date notices, suitable reading material and comfortable chairs. Clients should not be kept waiting for long periods and if any unavoidable delay occurs, receptionists need to ensure that clients are kept informed and not forgotten. Much will depend on the skill and aptitude of the reception staff to create a good first impression and appropriate training is essential.

Unobtrusive alarm systems also need to be sited in the reception areas and interview rooms and a co-ordinated response system should be available.

Daycare and residential settings

All the guidelines for avoiding violence in domestic and office settings apply equally to residential and daycare settings. However, there are a number of additional factors to be taken into account for dealing with larger numbers of people on one site. Making members feel it is their centre will go a long way to create an accepting atmosphere. Rules can usually be kept to a minimum, although most centres would want to forbid alcohol or drugs on the premises. Furthermore, good support and liaison with outside agencies adds strength to tackling individual problems.

However, the key to success is usually having adequate staffing ratios. Wiener (1983) makes the point that if there are too few staff around, it is impossible to identify all the clients who are having difficulties, so clients who want help have to create problems in order to attract staff attention. If too few staff are around, the centre becomes less safe for members. In relation to daycare, if too many members are in on any one day or if too many members are accepted over a short period of time, there are too many strangers in the centre for it to feel like a community of supportive friends.

Interview settings

Care should be taken with the physical layout of interview rooms. In the office setting it should be possible to arrange the seating and access to the door in a way that minimizes the risk of precipitous attack. In a domestic setting this is not always the case. However, where possible, try to survey the interview setting beforehand and remove any objects that could be used as a weapon, such as heavy glass ashtrays, ornaments, etc. A coffee table placed between the worker and the client keeps the former out of reach of a sudden swinging blow or lunge. Sitting close to an open door gives an opportunity for a hasty retreat and enables others to assist quickly if required. Meanwhile, sitting the client in a deep armchair means that he is less likely to be assaultive from a semi-recumbent position.

Interview method

Talking is probably the most effective way to help a client gain self-control so it is important that the interview is conducted in a calm and confident manner. The worker should adopt a professional, friendly approach. Violence is often precipitated by an anxious, insecure person or a domineering, authoritarian member of staff. While needing to be alert to the signs of violent behaviour, it is a mistake to treat the client as if he is dangerous as this can produce the reaction that the worker is seeking to avoid. At the same time, it is important to be aware of body posture and position and try to stand or sit in a way that will be least threatening to the client. The worker should be open and honest with the client and avoid whispering asides to colleagues. This is particularly relevant for the deaf, suspicious or paranoid client who may act adversely to vague or incorrect information.

Transporting clients

If there is thought to be the risk of violence, it is suggested that it would be inappropriate to transport the client by car. Although initially compliant, he may become disturbed or difficult during the journey. If a private car has to be used, the client should be seated in the rear behind the passenger seat with an escort. Child locks should also be activated to ensure that the client does not try to get out of the car while it is moving. Normally, where violence was anticipated, it would be necessary to seek assistance from the ambulance service and/or the police.

Physical intervention

Whenever possible, staff should retreat in the face of physical violence or threats. The first course of action should be to call for assistance either verbally or by use of an alarm system. Only if the client is about to be a danger to himself or others is physical intervention justified, with physical restraint being used only as a last resort. While all staff would benefit from the acquisition of breakaway skills, restraint techniques require practice and co-ordination with a minimum of three staff to avoid injury to themselves or the client. The use of physical restraint to repel violence is, in law, perfectly acceptable, subject to the qualification that 'restraint must only entail reasonable force'. 'Reasonable' means the amount of force that is sufficient to stop the attacker or to prevent yourself being injured. It should not be greater.

CLIENT'S RISK TO SELF

As a group, mentally disordered offenders pose a high risk of suicide and self-harm. Many possess a number of features associated with this type of behaviour and present a serious challenge for all professionals involved in their care. Typically, areas of the country that attract high rates of crime also attract high rates of suicidal behaviour though the link may be regarded as tenuous and more to do with an area being associated with social disorganization and abuse of alcohol and drugs. Nevertheless, the lifestyle and problems encountered by the mentally disordered offender often closely match the characteristics found in suicide-prone individuals.

Vaughan (1985) divides suicide-prone individuals into two groups: those with a relatively stable background who are overwhelmed by a social disaster and who lack the support or personal capacity to cope with the outcome, and those whose lives are marked by psychological instability and social disruption which is in evidence for many years before their fatal act. It is within this second group that many mentally disordered offenders fall, especially those brought before the Court for petty offences and who are now increasingly benefiting from diversion-to-treatment schemes. They are generally well-known to the psychiatric services, often having made previous attempts at suicide and having received in-patient treatment. A history of alcohol and/or drug abuse is common and their lifestyle is generally disorganized with multiple social problems.

They also form a small subgroup of chronic repeaters of deliberate self-harm. Unfortunately, they frequently respond poorly to any help offered, often rejecting attempts to bring order into their lives. Deliberate self-harm is often simply another way of seeking attention or gaining temporary relief from their troubles. Not surprisingly, such individuals alienate family and friends and become socially isolated and friendless.

Those who commit serious offences, however, tend to be at risk for different reasons. There is a small subsection of offenders who commit suicide at the time of their offence, not untypically, murder followed by suicide, often in the context of a psychotic depression. Sexual deviants may kill themselves in the course of the deviant act or in response to guilt or fear of exposure. The aftermath of committing a crime may itself be significant. Sainsbury (1955) found that in his sample of cases, where police action was pending, this was considered a contributory factor to suicide in 6% of cases. Prison suicides have risen dramatically in recent years, particularly in the remand population. It is argued that as well as the contributory factors of overcrowding leading to less supervision and support, prisons contain an excess of men with known risk factors for suicide such as previous psychiatric history, self-injury, alcohol or drug misuse, social isolation and marital disruption (Charlton *et al.*, 1993).

Those leaving hospital or prison may find reintegration into the community particularly difficult. The prejudice of potential employers and landlords is likely to severely hamper finding work or accommodation, leading to increasing feelings of rejection and isolation. As acute psychiatric illness is the most prominent factor immediately preceding suicide, the re-emergence of symptomatology particularly of depression or schizophrenia needs to be taken seriously. In her study over a four-year period of a group of 588 men who left Broadmoor, Norris (1984) found them to be significantly more at risk of suicide than those left behind. Of the 36 deaths that occurred in Broadmoor during this period, six (17%) died from unnatural causes. Of the 39 deaths that occurred in the discharged group over the same period 21 (54%) died from unnatural causes: 20 suicides and one murder. We can speculate on the pressures on the discharged group; their need for careful supervision and support is discussed more fully in Chapter Five.

Intervention

The government has set a target to reduce the suicide rate of severely mentally ill people by at least 33% by the year 2000 (D of H, 1993). Mentally disordered offenders are a particularly vulnerable group and where a risk of suicidal behaviour is thought to be present, active steps need to be taken to assess the level of risk and whether intervention is necessary. As with any other predictor of violent behaviour, suicide risk is best assessed by gathering as much relevant background information as possible. This will need to be supplemented by knowledge of the current situation faced by the client and an assessment of his current mental state. The following information may be particularly helpful:

- Family background and support: a disorganized family background often leads to a disorganized lifestyle in adulthood and increases the chances of irresponsible behaviour, including suicidal gestures. An unsympathetic or absent current family group contributes further to the risk of self-destructive behaviour. For example, single people are more vulnerable than those who are married and suicide is three times more common among divorced people than among those with partners.

- Personality: many people who attract the label of 'psychopath' or 'personality disorder' often give concern because of their self-destructive tendencies. Those with a criminal record, especially involving anti-social or aggressive behaviour, are more likely to engage in deliberate self-harm. Some who find themselves in a multitude of troubles use such action as a way of avoiding further responsibilities. The abuse of alcohol and/or drugs further increases the risk.
- Psychiatric illness: one of the biggest contributions to the suicide statistics is the presence of a formal mental illness, particularly depression and schizophrenia. People who have received in-patient and/or out-patient psychiatric treatment are more likely to make a suicide bid in times of distress.
- Previous suicide attempt: it is important to discover how a person usually deals with a crisis in order to gain some measure of his coping abilities. A previous suicidal gesture should always be treated seriously, as this certainly increases the likelihood of a subsequent attempt.
- Current problems: a catalogue of recent negative life events are likely to heighten the risk in vulnerable individuals, particularly those involving loss, social isolation and unemployment.

Having gained some understanding of the client's background and reasons for his current emotional state, the worker should have a rough idea of whether the client is at risk of harming himself. It will be apparent that the more features highlighted above which are present in an individual's situation, the greater the risk of self-harm. There are also a number of 'predictions of intent' and 'predictions of risk' scales that can be employed to assist in the process. A simple list devised by Buglass and Horton (1974) has proved fairly reliable in predicting whether somebody who has already harmed themselves will be at short-term risk of a further suicide attempt. They produced the following simple check list:

1. sociopathy;
2. problems with the use of alcohol;
3. previous in-patient psychiatric treatment;
4. previous out-patient psychiatric treatment;

5. previous deliberate self-harm resulting in hospital admission;
6. not living with a relative.

One point is scored for each characteristic present. It was found that the range of probability of repetition is 5% for a score of zero and up to 48% for a score of five or six. A further aid to assessing risk can be found by reference to the model developed by Vaughan (1984), illustrated in Figure 4.2. The model places vulnerable clients on a hierarchy of risk and is used as a framework for gaining some perspective on the presenting situation. The aim is to match the client's circumstances and presentation to an appropriate step on the model, with each step representing a distinct stage of risk; the higher the step, the greater the risk. It is possible to jump from the bottom to the top of the hierarchy due to mischance, but on the whole it should be possible to match the client to an appropriate level.

Having decided that a risk of suicide is present, it is necessary to decide the level of intervention needed to safeguard the situaiton. A useful techique described by Drye *et al.* (1973) is to share the evaluation of risk with the client and in doing so lessen the burden on the worker. It is suggested that the client himself is the best judge of how strong his urge is to end his life, and also how good his controls are. In other words, the client is in the best position to tell the worker how long and under what conditons he trusts himself to exercise control over his destructive impulses. Whenever the issue of suicide risk is being considered, the client should be asked whether he can honestly make the following statement: 'No matter what happens I will not kill myself accidentally or on purpose at any time.'

Drye and his colleagues go on to say that 'if the patient reports a feeling of confidence in this statement with no direct or indirect qualifications and with no incongruous voice tones or bodily movements, the evaluator may dismiss suicide as a management problem.' If such an assurance cannot be made, an element of risk is clearly present and the matter should be discussed at greater length. The researchers report a virtual 100% success rate

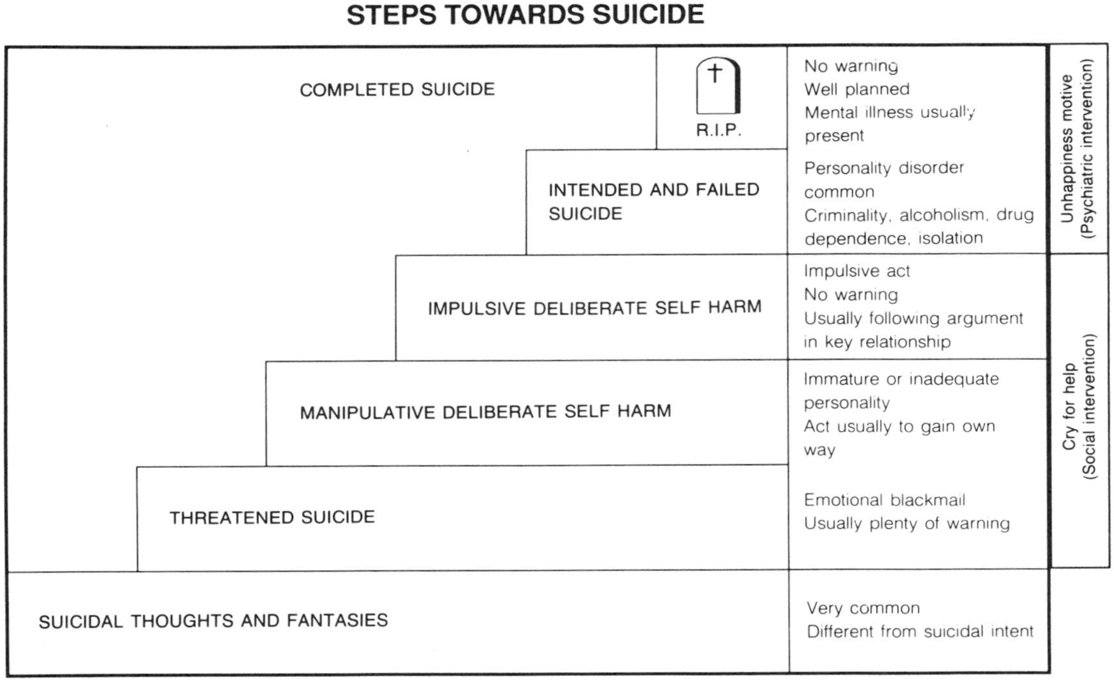

STEPS TOWARDS SUICIDE

Unhappiness motive (Psychiatric intervention)

Cry for help (Social intervention)

COMPLETED SUICIDE — R.I.P.

INTENDED AND FAILED SUICIDE
- No warning
- Well planned
- Mental illness usually present
- Personality disorder common
- Criminality, alcoholism, drug dependence, isolation

IMPULSIVE DELIBERATE SELF HARM
- Impulsive act
- No warning
- Usually following argument in key relationship

MANIPULATIVE DELIBERATE SELF HARM
- Immature or inadequate personality
- Act usually to gain own way

THREATENED SUICIDE
- Emotional blackmail
- Usually plenty of warning

SUICIDAL THOUGHTS AND FANTASIES
- Very common
- Different from suicidal intent

Figure 4.2 Steps towards suicide. (Adapted with permission from Vaughan, P.J. (1984) Steps towards suicide. *Community Care*, July 26, 14–16.)

in using this technique in the USA and they advocate its general application to clients with the exception of those with organic impairment, some psychotics and those who use alcohol and drugs heavily.

However, in some situations it will not be possible to obtain the client's reassurance that they will not harm themselves and a more active type of intervention will be necessary. At such times it is important for the worker to avoid being vague or woolly. The client will have more confidence in someone who does not flounder around but appears to have a clear plan of action. This is particularly important at a time when the client is confused or feeling helpless – and if suicide is imminent there is no room for hestitation or indecision.

Where the risk is considered slight, it may be enough to help the client ventilate his suicidal feelings and tackle any social and interpersonal problems. If the risk seems strong, frequent contact and close supervision will be required, together with a psychiatric assessment if a mental illness is apparent. This may in turn lead to admission to hospital in some cases. Where the risk is certain or imminent then the worker has no choice but to purposefully intervene. This may entail removing potential dangers such as drugs, car keys, etc., and accompanying the client until appropriate help is available. Mental illness is usually present in these circumstances and admission to hospital invariably follows either on a voluntary basis or under a section of the Mental Health Act 1983. A fuller account of the stages of suicidal behaviour and corresponding intervention can be found in *Suicide Prevention* by Vaughan (1985).

Finally the worker should, above all, communicate his concerns to others involved in the client's care in order to produce a co-ordinated and effective response to risk.

SUMMARY

Workers based in the community are inevitably placed at risk on occasions. Such risk may be exaggerated by work with mentally disordered offenders who may be more voltatile than other clients and may even have previously demonstrated their violent potential by aggressive behaviour or a violent crime.

Much care is needed in assessing the risk of each encounter and workers must consider the personal and situational factors leading to aggressive behaviour that are unique to each individual. This will involve a careful analysis of the client's background together with a methodical dissection of information about any previous incidents of violence. Such analysis should also include consideration of the likelihood of self as a target.

Of crucial importance is the sharing of information both within and across agencies to ensure that all who are involved with the client act in a cohesive way. Finally, where a potentially dangerous situation is identified, the worker must not shrink away from taking positive action to eliminate the risk. This may involve active support, aggressive outreach or the client's temporary removal to a safe place.

REFERENCES

Breakwell, G. (1989) *Facing Physical Violence*, British Psychological Society, Leicester.

Brown, R., Bute, S. and Ford, P. (1986) *Social Workers at Risk: the Prevention and Management of Violence*, Macmillan Education, Basingstoke.

Buglass, D. and Horton, J. (1974) A scale for predicting subsequent suicidal behaviour. *British Journal of Psychiatry*, **124**, 573–8.

Bute, S. (1979) Guidelines for coping with violence by clients. *Social Work Today*, Vol. II, **15**, 13–14.

Charlton, J. Kelly, S., Dunnell, K., Evans, B. and Jenkins, R. (1993) Suicide deaths in England and Wales: trends in factors associated with suicide deaths. *Population Trends*, Spring, **71**, 34–42.

Department of Health (1993) *The Health of the Nation, Key Area Handbook: Mental Illness* HMSO, London.

Department of Health and Social Security (1988) *Report of the Committee of Inquiry into the Care and After-Care of Miss Sharon Campbell*, Cmnd 440, HMSO, London.

Dryer, R.C., Goulding, R.L. and Goulding, M.E. (1973) No suicide decisions: patient monitoring of suicide risk. *American Journal of Psychiatry*, **130**, 171–4.

Health Services Advisory Committee (1987) *Violence to Staff in the Health Services*, Health and Safety Executive, HMSO, London.

Monahan, J. (1981) *Predicting Violent Behaviour*, Sage Publications, Beverly Hills.

Norris, M. (1984) *Integration of Special Hospital Patients into the Community*, Gower Publishing, Aldershot.

Prins, H. (1986) *Dangerous Behaviour the Law and Mental Disorder*, Tavistock, London.

Ritchie, J.H., Dick, D. and Lingham, R. (1994) *The Report of the Inquiry into the Care and Treatment of Christopher Clunis*, Presented to the Chairman of North East Thames and South East Thames Regional Health Authorities, HMSO, London.

Rowett, C. (1986) *Violence in Social Work*, Institute of Criminology, Occasional paper No. 14, Cambridge University, Cambridge.

Sainsbury, P. (1955) *Suicide in London*, Maudsley Monograph, No. 1, Chapman & Hall, London.

Scott, P.D. (1977) Assessing dangerousness in criminals. *British Journal of Psychiatry*, **131**, 127–42.

Stenge, L.R. (1977) *The Prevention and Management of Disturbed Behaviour*, Ministry of Health, Ontario.

Vaughan, P.J. (1984) Steps towards suicide. *Community Care*, 26 July, 14–16.

Vaughan, P.J. (1985) *Suicide Prevention*, Pepar Publications, Birmingham.

Vaughan, P.J. (1988) Management of the compulsory psychiatric admission. *Community Psychiatry*, Vol. 1., No. 1, 5–6.

Weiner, R. (1983) When emotions overflow. *Community Care*, 14 April, 16–17.

5

Primary and secondary prevention

Most of this chapter is devoted to a discussion of the application of government directives, policies and legislative measures targeted at those clearly identified as mentally disordered offenders. However, the first part seeks to extend the discussion about 'invisible' and unrecognized mentally disordered offenders begun in Chapter One. The aim is to stimulate a wide range of professionals to consider if they might have people such as this on their caseloads. The proposal is that a recognition of such cases would be helpful to the individual clients, their families and carers, as well as to the worker. It will also be argued that such recognition also provides greater safeguards for the general public.

WHAT IS PRIMARY PREVENTION?

The notions of primary, secondary and tertiary prevention come from the field of public health where they have been successfully applied in tackling and in some cases eliminating disease. Primary prevention is directed at populations that are considered to be at risk of developing disease in the future, secondary prevention with the early detection and treatment of disease, while tertiary prevention, broadly speaking, is rehabilitation aimed at preventing further deterioration among those who have already suffered illness. In ethical terms there are few problems with either secondary or tertiary prevention as both are focused on identified patients who have symptoms for which they will probably want treatment. However, primary prevention involves interventions with healthy populations in order to prevent some ill occurring in the future. For such a measure to be accepted there needs to be some consensus that it will prevent the predicted ill and that the risks of becoming ill in the future substantially outweigh any risks connected with the intervention. The fluoridation of water is an example of a measure where there was dispute on both counts.

Translating this schema to the field of mentally disordered offenders, it is not hard to see the social supervision of those on Restriction Orders as coming under the heading of tertiary prevention. The goal of the social supervisor is to rehabilitate the offender-patient and to monitor his progress in the community so that he does not deteriorate and become a danger to himself or others. Secondary prevention is covered in the latter stages of the chapter where divert-to-treatment and care management can both be seen to fit comfortably within an overall aim of early identification of need in order to make interventions that are designed to minimize the number and length of admissions to institutional care. It is hard to see any general ethical problems with this type of intervention, though individual cases may well provide dilemmas about the balance between care and control responsibilities.

The question about what constitutes primary prevention in relation to community care of the mentally disordered offender, however, is not quite so clear. The burden of the argument in Chapter One was that there are a number of at-risk populations that should be considered for primary prevention measures. These are known offenders both in custody and under supervision in the community, persons known to be mentally disordered and under the care and supervision of mental health professionals and finally those known and under the care of health and welfare workers but whose mental health needs and potential and/or actual offending are not currently recognized or acted upon.

Looking at those in the criminal justice system first, it seems that there is strong support in some quarters for what might be called primary prevention measures. For example, it is widely recognized that the way prisons are built, staffed and managed has a major effect on the mental health of the inmates. This has dramatic confirmation when prisoners run riot and destroy the premises. There is less dramatic confirmation when young offenders commit suicide, though the link to mental health issues is perhaps clearer in these sad cases. The fact that such an analysis commands wide support among informed professionals, including Judge Tumin, the Chief Inspector of Prisons, does not mean that this will be accepted as government policy and at the time of writing the current Home Secretary, Michael Howard, seems committed to measures that will increase overcrowding in prisons and make regimes more punitive. Such measures, if implemented, are likely both to increase the number of offenders who become mentally disordered and reduce the help available to them.

However, the same government is not totally against the idea of the primary prevention of crime as was revealed by the reported enthusiasm of one minister for identifying those young children with a propensity to commit offences in later life. The approach being advocated was not one of general preventive measures, such as increased numbers of nursery classes, youth clubs and job-creation schemes, but targeted interventions directed towards at-risk individuals. These proposals demonstrate a new-found confidence in the capacity of the social sciences to identify at-risk individuals and in social workers and probation officers to intervene effectively with them once identified. It will be evident from this brief discussion that any primary prevention measure must be based on a model or theory of causation. Not surprisingly, there is as much dispute about such theories as there is about any other model of human behaviour and given the timescale for primary prevention even less chance of resolving disputes by appeals to the evidence. In such a situation it is important to proceed cautiously and only to implement policies that command general support.

Moving to the second group, that of known persons suffering from mental disorder, the questions are whether it is possible or desirable to identify who is at risk of offending and whether any particular preventive intervention is likely to be effective. In general terms the big risk is of further stigmatizing those with mental disorders by even raising the possibility that they might also be offenders. The general public may already tend to believe in such an association and it is important not to reinforce such misconceptions. Equally it could be experienced as very demoralizing to individual patients and clients if community psychiatric nurses and social workers were routinely to start raising questions with individuals about the possibility that they were committing offences.

A counter-argument is that mental health workers owe a duty to their clients, the clients' families and carers, and to the general public wherever possible to prevent crime, particularly crimes of violence. The argument being advanced is similar to the one that obtains in relation to child protection: namely, that there is little merit in waiting for someone to be damaged before intervening. The whole point of being involved is to prevent such damage occurring, whether it is self-harm or violence towards others. Until quite recently the research evidence suggested both that the mentally disordered were no more likely than others to commit dangerous offences and that psychiatrists and others were likely to overpredict violence rather than underestimate it (Steadman and Cocozza, 1974). However, the association between mental disorder and offending which has been observed at a clinical level is now finding confirmation in research. Hodgins' recent review (1993) provides a helpful and informative summary of both the evidence and the methodological difficulties associated with such research. Not all those suffering from a mental disorder are at a higher-than-average risk of offending but those that combine a diagnosis of a major mental disorder, alcohol and drug abuse are at high risk. There will probably be different rates of association for different diagnoses. It does seem that there is sufficient evidence to warrant professional energy being put into preventive strategies.

How then is a practitioner to weigh up the situation and to find a satisfactory way forward? The modest and manageable first step is to focus on existing caseloads and to identify which people are at risk of offending and in what ways. This is likely to leave a large number of individuals who are not considered to be at risk and can therefore be removed from the target population for any preventive measures. Of those at risk, priority should be given to those where offences against the person are a major concern. Grounds for putting someone in this category would include those with a history of such behaviour (whether it had led to criminal charges or not) and threats of such behaviour. It may seem excessive to include the latter but much as with threats of suicide it is prudent to believe people when they say they intend to hurt someone. It may also be of interest that the Tarasoff ruling (Barker and Branson, 1993) in the Supreme Court of California in July 1976 laid a 'duty to warn' on therapists whose clients uttered threats against others during counselling. Though there is no legal equivalent in the UK this ruling provides a timely reminder that mental health professionals have a duty to potential victims as well as to their clients.

For those working with people who have a history of violence towards others, it is important to bear in mind this propensity towards violence at all stages of their work. There is a good case for having a system of marking files so that new workers in particular do not miss this crucial information because it is buried in the depths of the file. As has been pointed out in Chapter Two, mental health provider units have been required since 1 April 1994, to establish a register of those patients considered at risk of serious violence to themselves or others. The civil liberties issues here are considerable but so are the safety of workers and others. Where the identified risk is of non-violent crime, such as theft, the issues of protection may well decrease and so measures such as marking files may not be needed. The prevention of nuisance crimes is much more likely to be achieved by attention to issues such as homelessness, poverty and restoration to a settled way of life. This requires the worker to give as much attention to clients and patients who are often portrayed as 'hopeless cases' as they give to others who perhaps have less overwhelming needs and are more likely to respond rapidly to the help offered.

For the mental health worker the big shift that a preventive approach to this client group requires is to encompassing the possibility that someone under their care may commit serious or petty offences *and* to accept the challenge of intervening to prevent this occurrence. This is not to say that every community psychiatric nurse and approved social worker should become a quasi-probation officer. However, such workers can learn from their probation colleagues the skills, knowledge and approach that allows offending behaviour to be on the agenda for both the worker and the client.

The final group – those who are known to health and welfare workers but whose mental disorder and offending behaviour are not officially recognized – raises the most issues in terms of the legitimacy and usefulness of a preventive approach. In some ways it could be portrayed as a Messianic endeavour to cast the net so wide that almost everyone and anyone could be considered to have the potential to be a mentally disordered offender. The intention is more modest and more serious. The concern is about those people who are currently known to general practitioners, CPNs and social workers who are a cause for concern but the nature of this concern has not been realized. Cohen and Fisher (1987) have demonstrated that both doctors and social workers have difficulty in recognizing mental health problems and this is probably also true for probation officers. It is not easy to be sure why these groups should have difficulty in identifying such problems, though lack of training is often advanced as a reason. A likely explanation is lack of experience in dealing with mental illness and, in the case of social workers, a diffidence about accepting that this is part of their job. If child care or care of older people is the focus of one's work, it may seem to be exceeding one's remit to tackle mental health problems too.

Accepting a mental health dimension to social work with other client groups is a big step and it may seem an even bigger one to also consider whether the individual is also offending or is likely to do so. In practice, it is likely that concern about the possibility of offences being committed will already have arisen. For example, in the field of domestic violence many social workers and health care professionals are only too aware of the risk that violent offences will be committed, usually by men on women and children. Until recently, the police were reluctant to intervene in this field and it could be said to be progress that charges will now be brought for offences committed within the home. So it can be seen that criminalizing behaviour can be a step forward because it means a problem has been recognized. However, it is in everyone's interests to act before such offences take place if this is at all possible. One method of prevention is for the potential victims to leave the family home. The growth in the number of refuges for women and children is clearly crucial for this strategy. Alternatively, legal measures can be taken to remove the offender from the home and prevent him from returning. A further alternative is offered where there are grounds for believing that the offender is mentally disordered and in such situations action under the 1983 Mental Health Act should be considered. Such a possibility will only be available if the social worker, refuge worker or the police have an understanding of mental disorder and how it relates to offending.

The common element in primary prevention with all three of these target populations is the awareness of the worker of the dimensions of mental disorder and offending behaviour so that when appropriate these may become part of the assessment of the person and their situation. It is also important that workers widen their concept of their professional area to encompass a responsibility for identifying potentially mentally disordered offenders and where possible intervening to prevent them committing offences. The final point of discussion before moving on to secondary prevention proper is to acknowledge that some of what is being advocated above teeters on the boundary between primary and secondary prevention. The design of prisons and remand centres is clearly primary prevention but identifying that a violent husband is mentally disordered is probably closer to early detection and becomes an example of secondary prevention. This probably does not matter if the broad thrust of this section has persuaded the reader of the value and importance of recognizing those who may become (and perhaps already are) mentally disordered offenders. Some may be persuaded of the arguments but remain sceptical about the value or effectiveness of psychiatric intervention.

Over the last 30 years, psychiatry has not had a particularly good press and many social workers will have devoted as much time in their training to the abuses of psychiatry as to its effectiveness. Equally, the dangers and side-effects of drugs prescribed by psychiatrists may have had more publicity than their usefulness in the management of those suffering from psychoses. The thrust of this book is not to disregard these concerns nor to set aside the important civil liberty issues that accompany the use of the Mental Health Act 1983. However, the general approach is a positive one in which the value of well-planned multidisciplinary interventions is assumed. It is not the case that a psychiatrist will always be the lead person because in the community most day-to-day responsibility is carried by CPNs, social workers, probation officers and the staff of residential and daycentres. Nevertheless, the importance for all these groups of having readily available and competent psychiatric advice is critical. Where others have questioned the right to intervene and the dangers of doing so, the approach that is being proposed assumes that there are far more dangers of this client group being neglected in the community and of late interventions resulting which are overly restrictive and non-therapeutic. Positive and early action is at the heart of both primary and secondary prevention and skills in this sort of work can go a long way to prevent panicky, heavy-end-interventions when the client has become seriously disordered and/or dangerous.

For those clients who become identified as mentally disordered offenders, a range of legal and policy frameworks are available to community-based workers to guide their intervention. These are discussed below.

DIVERSION FROM CUSTODY

For some years there has been concern that too many mentally ill and vulnerable people are inappropriately held in prison. Unnecessary involvement in the criminal justice system is not only an expensive and inefficient response to their needs but is also likely to cause further damage and deterioration to their mental health. Sone (1990) gives an example of how the criminal justice system continues to fail this group of offenders:

Case study

Jeffrey Rofe, a 25-year-old New Zealander, arrived in London in May 1989 to start a two-year working holiday. On 17 June 1990 he was arrested for burning pages from his address book. Ten weeks later he was found dead on his cell floor in Brixton prison after strangling himself with a shirt sleeve. Rofe's crime was to suffer from paranoid schizophrenia. His tragedy was to get caught up in a criminal justice system that consistently fails those suffering from mental illness.

It was because of such tragic failures of the system, together with the concern over the large numbers of mentally disordered people in prison generally, that prompted the government to consider ways of tackling the problem. This led directly to the issuing of Home Office Circular 66/90 which drew the attention of those working in the criminal justice system to the existing legal powers for dealing with mentally disordered offenders and encouraged effective inter-agency co-operation to promote the diversion of the mentally disordered to the health and social services (Home Office, 1990). It stated that the mentally disordered should not be drawn into the criminal justice system because of their disorder, for example in the hope of securing treatment in the Prison Health Care System. These directives were subsequently endorsed by the Reed Report which included such developments in its recommendations (D of H/HO, 1992).

Within two years of issuing Home Office Circular 66/90 it is reported that about 60 diversion schemes had been developed with more in the planning stage (Home Office, 1993). There is no single model for such schemes nor any dictate as to who should be involved, as it is intended that schemes should reflect local needs and working practices. Accordingly, there is a great variety in the schemes that have been developed, ranging from single part-time workers providing a limited service to the Courts to multi-disciplinary teams providing a sophisticated specialist service.

Diversion from custody can take place at any decision point in the criminal justice system but ideally it should occur as early as possible in the process. The role of the worker in the divert scheme is to assist and advise those who have the authority to make such decisions and to facilitate any subsequent support necessary for the client. The choice points and options available are illustrated in Table 5.1.

As an example of how a well co-ordinated service can function it is worth quoting an extract from a briefing paper of the Diversion from Custody Project in Hull (North Humberside MIND, 1993):

1. The team
    The project is based in the central offices of North Humberside MIND. The Project Team is made up of an approved social worker, a community psychiatric nurse and a probation officer. Together they seek to achieve the aims of the project by intervening at every decision-making point in

the criminal justice system to enable non-custodial disposals to be made.

2. The day
    The team start their day at 7.30 a.m. by visiting each of the three Hull police stations in order to identify and assess any mentally disordered offenders in custody, at the earliest point possible in the criminal system. The team liaise with custody officers to facilitate diversion, where possible.

3. The work
    At 8.45 a.m. the team meet at Hull Magistrates' court where they pool information on their separate visits to the police stations. They then assess prisoners in the court cells, decide priorities and allocate work in the courts. By 9.30 a.m. they are ready to consult with the Crown Prosecution and defence solicitors. They offer advice and information and will make arrangements for appropriate housing or bail support to avoid the necessity of a remand or sentence to custody. Each team member then follows through his individual carework during the court day. They may be called to give evidence that a particular defendant is known to the project and that they will make arrangements for that person as the Court considers necessary in order to grant bail. One team member has special responsibility for liaising with prison staff and taking referrals from HM Prison, Hull and the Wolds Remand Prison. The team meet up at the end of the day in their own office to exchange information and to plan for the following day. They work together collectively and collaboratively, pooling their individual knowledge and expertise to provide a responsive and effective service.

The team is supported by a rota of psychiatrists on one morning each week to carry out psychiatric assessments. Where a non-custodial disposal is effected, referral is made to the local community mental health teams for continued support.

There are now many examples of the above schemes throughout the country involving workers of all disciplines. However, despite some funding initiatives created by the Home Office many are dependent on short-term grants or local funding arrangements. Without long-term secure funding,

Table 5.1 Procedures available to effect divergence to treatment and discontinuance from prosecution

Stage one: at the police station	
(i)	After removal to a place of safety (preferably a hospital) under Section 136 of the Mental Health Act 1983 a mental health assessment should be arranged which will have the following range of disposal options: – Informal admission to hospital – Section 2 or 3 MHA '83 (compulsory admission to hospital) – Section 7 MHA '83 (admission to Guardianship) – Informal support in the Community – No further action
(ii)	Where an offence is suspected to have been committed but it appears that prosecution is not required a caution may be given or any of the above options used
(iii)	Where an offence is suspected to have been committed and it is decided to investigate further, the following action should be taken: – examination by the forensic medical examiner – person to be interviewed in the presence of an appropriate' adult under section 66 of the Police and Criminal Evidence Act 1984
(iv)	Where a prosecution is pursued bail facilities to be sought at an appropriate hostel or hospital
(v)	After a charge is made a multi-agency assessment should be arranged to ensure any necessary treatment is given and to advise the Court on disposal
Stage two: in court	
(i)	As an alternative to imposing a prison sentence the Magistrates' Court may make the following orders: – Section 35 MHA '83 (remand to hospital for assessment) – Section 37 MHA '83 (Hospital Order) – Section 37 MHA '83 (Guardianship Order) – Section 38 MHA '83 (Interim hospital order) – Probation Order with a condition of psychiatric treatment – Conditional discharge – Absolute discharge
(ii)	As an alternative to imposing a prison sentence the Crown Court may make the following orders: – All of the above made by the Magistrates' court – Section 36 MHA '83 (remand to hospital for treatment) – Section 41 MHA '83 (Restriction Order)

Table 5.1 *contd*

Additionally in cases where the accused is found to be unfit to plead under the Criminal Procedures (Insanity and Unfitness to Plead) Act 1991 the following diposal options are available:
- Hospital Order (with or without restrictions)
- Guardianship Order
- Supervision and Treatment Order
- Absolute discharge

Stage three: in prison

Prison medical officers should where they consider it appropriate recommend the following:
- Section 47 MHA '83 (Transfer to hospital for treatment sentenced prisoner)
- Section 48 MHA '83 (Transfer to hospital for treatment remand prisoner

some of the schemes may face discontinuance themselves. Already some projects, despite their success, have 'been lost or shelved due to lack of funding, or in some cases lack of commitment from key agencies' (National Practitioners Group, 1993).

PSYCHIATRIC/PANEL ASSESSMENT SCHEMES

Traditionally, many homeless mentally ill petty offenders have been remanded into custody for psychiatric assessment following their initial court appearance. The use of prison for this purpose is determined by the offender's lack of community ties and the absence of adequate bail hostels. The result has been lengthy and unnecessary detention in prison simply for the purpose of obtaining a medical report, with the irony that few offenders subsequently go to hospital (Bowden, 1978).

A much-quoted scheme designed to overcome these difficulties is one described by Joseph and Potter (1990). Theirs is a report of a research study on a service established at the Inner London Magistrates Courts of Bow Street and Marlborough Street, which has transferred the focus of assessment from the prison to the magistrates court. A psychiatrist is available for two sessions per week to receive referrals from magistrates, probation officers, duty solicitors and police officers, to assess those appearing in court for the first time following arrest and those remanded in custody for psychiatric reports. By undertaking the assessment at the court, the psychiatrist has much better access to relevant records, personnel, etc. It also facilitates direct discussion with the Crown Prosecution Service with a view to discontinuance and appropriate disposal. The study showed that a rate of 35% discontinuance was achieved by these schemes compared to the usual rate of 1%–2%.

Annex C of Home Office Circular 66/90 described an extension to this approach involving a multi-agency assessment panel. It drew on the experience of the Hertfordshire Panel Assessment Scheme which was established in 1985 with the purpose of co-ordinating the contributions of various agencies involved in preparing reports on an accused person's mental state and the availability of hospital accommodation or community care. The circular itself encourages the development of such schemes wherever possible. The original concept was that a panel would be convened following a referral from the court for a psychiatric and social assessment. By sharing professional opinion and agreeing appropriate use of resources it avoided the court receiving pre-sentence and psychiatric reports which contained conflicting recommendations. Furthermore, the multi-agency approach ensured shared responsibility and co-ordination of response, should a community disposal be made.

The composition of the panels will vary with each scheme but apart from the co-ordinator, who may be of any discipline, it will include a psychiatrist and probation officer together with any combination of community psychiatric nurse, social worker, GP, housing officer, employer, etc. Many schemes now meet when required by the Court as above but also at the request of either the police or Crown Prosecution Service before Court when cautioning or discontinuance is considered. They may also be used during statutory supervision, or before and after discharge from hospital, regional secure unit or prison.

It should be added that many panels are loosely formed and do not always meet on a regular formal basis. In many instances, the co-ordinator bears the brunt of the work, often holding telephone conferences as a way of speeding up what may be a difficult and time-consuming task of assembling everybody together on a frequent basis.

A recent evaluation of three different panel-assessment schemes commissioned by the Home Office revealed considerable variety in their working and membership and concludes that it is not possible to construct a blueprint for the ideal scheme (Hedderman, 1993). However, a number of common features were identified as key elements:

1. All agencies involved must make an initial commitment, including a willingness to allocate resources needed to make the scheme work;
2. a steering group is needed from the outset to give a sense of joint ownership of the project, common purpose and a vested interest in seeing the arrangements succeed;
3. membership of the group must be at senior level to be able to implement agreed policies; and
4. arrangements must be set up to monitor and evaluate the scheme.

ACTING AS AN 'APPROPRIATE ADULT' UNDER THE POLICE AND CRIMINAL EVIDENCE ACT 1984

On 1 April 1991 a revised Code of Practice came into effect in respect of Section 66 of the Police and Criminal Evidence Act 1984 (Home Office, 1991). It recognized that although persons who are mentally disordered or mentally handicapped are often capable of providing reliable evidence, they may also without knowing or wishing to do so, be particularly prone in certain circumstances to provide information that is unreliable, misleading or self-incriminating. Special care therefore should always be exercised in questioning such a person and an appropriate adult should be involved if there is any doubt about a person's mental state or capacity.

The Code states that if a police officer suspects or is told in good faith that a person is suffering from a mental disorder or is mentally handicapped, or mentally incapable of understanding the significance of questions put to her/him, then that person shall be treated as a mentally disordered or mentally handicapped person for the purposes of the Code.

Accordingly a person who fulfils this criteria, whether suspected or not, must not be interviewed or asked to provide or sign a written statement in the absence of an appropriate adult apart only for exceptional cases (defined in Annex C of the Code).

In this context an 'appropriate adult' means:

1. a relative, guardian or other person responsible for his/her care or custody;
2. someone who has experience of dealing with mentally disordered or mentally handicapped persons but is not a police officer or employed by the police (such as an approved social worker or specialist social worker); or
3. failing either of the above, some other responsible adult aged 18 or over who is not a police officer or employed by the police.

The implementation of the above process will vary according to local arrangements. In some cases, clear policies have been developed between the police and local social services departments identifying the process for gaining access to an appropriate adult. Some agencies have commissioned trained volunteers to act in this capacity. In other areas *ad hoc* arrangements exist and the police are often left to seek out a willing appropriate adult themselves. Finding an appropriate adult, particularly in the middle of the night, is not always an easy task and the first step in implementing the Codes of Practice should be the development of a local policy for each police area which identifies the appropriate first contact point for the custody officer. Whichever agency or person is designated to respond to a request from the custody officer to attend the police station, in the capacity of an appropriate adult, should have a clear understanding of the process involved. This is described under the following headings:

The referral

On receiving a referral from the custody officer, information about the circumstances surrounding the arrest need to be sought, such as is the person a volunteer? has he been arrested? at what time was he detained? what is the reason for the arrest or detention? At this stage it is also worth ascertaining whether the person has any communication difficulties and is in need of a trained interpreter so that the necessary arrangements can be put in hand if needed. Having gathered the relevant preliminary information, the police need to be advised of the appropriate adult's expected time of arrival which should be recorded in the custody record.

Careful thought needs to be given as to who should actually carry out the role of the appropriate adult. The Code notes that for persons 'who are mentally disordered or mentally handicapped it may in certain circumstances be more satisfactory for all concerned if the appropriate adult is someone who has experience or training in their care rather than a relative lacking in such qualifications. But if the person himself prefers a relative to a better qualified stranger his wishes should, if practicable, be respected.' This would seem to indicate a preference for a mental health professional from the local community mental health or learning disabilities team, or perhaps a relevant residential or daycare worker who knows the client. Even so, it has to be borne in mind that police stations can be intimidating places. The so-called 'liberal' attitudes of social workers are not always welcome in what is essentially a 'macho' culture. Female staff may feel particularly uncomfortable. It is advisable therefore that only experienced, qualified and trained workers who are prepared for the task are used. Needless to say, it is also desirable to try to match the worker with the client in terms of gender, race, colour, language, etc.

Notwithstanding the above there are some workers who are specifically barred from acting in this capacity, other than the police or those employed by the police. These are:

- a solicitor who is present at the police station in a professional capacity may not act as the appropriate adult (Code C, Note 1F);
- a probation officer cannot act in this capacity (R.V. O'Neill, Birmingham Crown Court, 1990);
- approved social workers are not legally barred from undertaking this task but the Home Office and Department of Health booklet on good practice states that 'It is important to recognise the potential conflict which may arise where an approved social worker is called in by the police to

make an assessment for the purposes of the Mental Health Act and is subsequently requested to perform the role of "appropriate adult" during an investigative interview. One person should not be asked to fulfil both functions unless the circumstances are exceptional.' (HO/D of H, 1993).

At the police station

Before the client is seen, a check should be made that he has been examined by the forensic medical examiner and that it has been confirmed that he is fit to be detained and fit to be interviewed. If this is confirmed the client should be seen on his own before the police interview takes place. The client can refuse to see the worker alone but on the other hand can insist on doing so if he wishes.

Once alone with the client, the worker should explain who he is and why he is there while ensuring that the client fully understands what is going on. A check should be made to see if he was informed of his rights on arrival at the police station and if he has been cautioned. Both will need to be repeated by the police in the worker's presence. Above all, the client should understand his right to free legal advice. Only if the case goes to court will there be a charge for legal help. If it is felt that the client is not making an informed choice and legal advice would be advisable, the worker can ask for a solicitor even if the client does not want one.

The client should not be engaged in any discussion about the alleged offence as the worker may not be bound by confidence if the client admits to the offence in the worker's presence. Finally, appropriate action may need to be taken if there are any complaints about inappropriate treatment in the police station which contravene the conditions for detention.

The police interview

The worker's presence in the police interview is to ensure that the interview is not carried out in an oppressive manner. This could cover the style of interviewing, physical intimidation, threats, nearness of face-to-face contact, etc. If at any point it is felt that the interview is getting out of hand the worker should inform the interviewer that he is not happy with the way the interview is being conducted. The worker may also act to facilitate communication where necessary, and if it is felt that the proceedings should be brought to a halt he can always choose to leave the room. This has the effect of automatically stopping the interview.

It is always important to take notes during the interview as these may be needed for reference if the worker is subsequently called to give evidence in court.

After the police interview

When the interview is over, the worker should remain with the client to witness any subsequent proceedings such as identification, finger-printing, photographing, cautioning, charging, etc. If the case is to be brought to court the worker should draw any concerns he may have to the defence solicitor and check on who will represent the client in court.

In conclusion, if there are no further police proceedings the worker should ensure that any property is returned and assistance is given to enable the client to return to the community.

CARE MANAGEMENT

The logical outcome of these measures must be an increase in the number of mentally disordered offenders who need care and support in the community. As prisons are used decreasingly as substitutes for bail hostels, psychiatric wards and hostels for the homeless, pressure must mount for community-based facilities of this type. Similarly, as diversion and panel-assessment schemes become increasingly successful, community services will be called upon more frequently. Offenders who would traditionally have spent short periods in prison or have been supported solely by the probation service are now being presented to a much wider range of professionals for community support.

Unfortunately, like the long-term mentally ill, mentally disordered offenders are not always greeted with open arms by mental health professionals who often prefer working with those who are more likely to progress and get better. A study of six new community mental health teams by Patmore and

Weaver (1992) showed that a powerful influence to the detriment of the long-term mentally ill was staff preference for clients without indicators of serious mental disorder. Mentally disordered offenders are not only likely to have a long-term mental illness but are also less likely to be compliant with care programmes even though they may have been diverted from custody by virtue of their agreement to such care. An added difficulty for the worker may be the need to take into account the welfare of others and the infringement of an unsympathetic public view on the care plan. Thus it is not surprising to hear that 'Anecdotal evidence seems to suggest that many vulnerable individuals placed in the "community" find themselves in quite unsupportive, even desperate, circumstances' (Watson, 1993).

If the mentally disordered offender is to be diverted away from custodial care, he needs a 'champion' in the community who is going to ensure that an individualized, flexible package of care is arranged to suit his needs. Shepherd (1993) claims that a care manager is the obvious candidate to co-ordinate the input from various agencies, provide consistency and commitment and act as an advocate on behalf of the client. The introduction of care management systems was discussed briefly here in Chapter Two under the heading NHS and Community Care Act 1990 and the use of care management in mental health is fully described by Onyett (1992).

The care manager can come from any profession but as the budget for packages of care are held by the local authority, the care manager will probably come from a social services team or a joint agency mental health team. Ideally, a representative of this team should be a member of any panel-assessment scheme in order to be able to commit team support and financial assistance to the care plan. However, where the client is already known to the probation service, a probation officer may well be better placed to fulfil this function and to act as a care manager on behalf of the local authority. The same would apply to other non-local authority employees such as a community psychiatric nurse.

One of the biggest drawbacks, however, is that budgetary constraints mean that the needs of the mentally disordered offender have to be considered alongside those of other client groups with the effect that the former often get lower priority.

Such difficulties have led NACRO's Mental Helth Advisory Committee to recommend that funding to local authorities from the Department of Health for community care provision should be ring-fenced with specific provision for the needs of mentally disordered offenders (NACRO Mental Health Advisory Committee, 1993). Care managers will therefore find themselves balancing the needs of their 'diverted' clients against those of their other equally needy clients.

The actual work undertaken will depend on the model of care management adopted by the particular local authority. Shepherd (1993) favours the 'clinical, casework model' which is more like the traditional role of the experienced probation officer or forensic psychiatrist where therapeutic long-term support and advice is given to the offender patient. The key to helping clients deal more effectively with their problems lies in developing a stable, consistent relationship. In effect the worker becomes both 'purchaser' and 'provider' for the client.

Conversely, some agencies are appointing care managers solely as 'brokers' of care. In this model it is often considered that the care manager need not be a professional at all as their function is more akin to an administrative manager. Where such systems exist, more reliance may need to be placed on the key worker within the Care Programme Approach. Indeed *The Health of the Nation* handbook on mental illness sees the two roles as distinct and complementary (D of H, 1993).

Whichever model is used, much will depend on inter-agency and inter-professional collaboration and co-operation. Moreover, as the mentally disordered offender tends not to make demands on the services they require, it is up to the care manager to do it for him.

PROBATION ORDER WITH A CONDITION OF PSYCHIATRIC TREATMENT

A community alternative to custody little used by the courts is the probation order with a condition of psychiatric treatment. It would appear to be ideally suited for those offenders with a mild form of mental illness and yet it does not appear to be a popular disposal option. In 1973 almost 200 orders were made as opposed to currently half that number. Remarkably little research has been carried out into their use and efficacy and the reason for the decrease in such orders over the last 20 years is not known.

The order can be made for a person convicted of any offence except murder and lasts between six months and three years. As well as requiring the offender to be under the supervision of a probation officer, certain conditions may be attached including residence at a specified place which may include a psychiatric hospital. Treatment may be either as an in-patient or an out-patient under the directiot of a named doctor. However, as the order can be made only if the offender consents, psychiatric treatment cannot be imposed against his will except under emergency conditions. If the place of residence is a psychiatric hospital, he is in effect an informal patient. Compulsory treatment against his will can be carried out only by making him subject to a relevant section of the Mental Health Act 1983.

In its simplest form, the order can help the mildly disordered petty offender by preventing repeated appearances in court. A case described by Major (1991) illustrates its application.

Case study

A man appeared in court charged with the theft of a Mars bar. He was a discharged mental patient and he said that he felt he was becoming ill again. He had asked for help but none was forthcoming, so he went into a newsagent, picked up a Mars bar, held it up and said 'I'm stealing this'.

The man was brought to court and remanded for a medical report. The report said he was fine when he took his medication but that he had neglected to get his medication from his GP. The magistrates wished to encourage this very minor offender to consult his GP on a regular basis and used the probation order with a condition of psychiatric treatment to enable a duly qualified medical practitioner to direct the patient to consult his GP.

In this case the order appears to have been used simply to ensure the offender had access to and used his GP. At the same time, he would have had the benefit of supervision from the probation officer. It could be argued, however, that the emerging divert schemes would make such a simple order unnecessary. A panel-assessment scheme would just as easily have established a community-support network and could even have avoided him coming to court in the first place.

Normally, orders are issued for more serious offences with offences against property and sexual offences being most commonly represented. Offenders suffering from depression, personality disorder and alcohol and drug dependence have also been considered suitable for such orders (Lewis, 1980). There is the added advantage that, after a period of hospitalization, there will be statutory provision of after-care unlike a Hospital Order without restriction (Section 37) which has no such mandatory follow-up.

For the probation officer the same responsibilities and obligations will apply as with a 'normal' probation order. The objectives are;

- to secure the rehabilitation of the offender;
- to protect the public from harm from the offender; and/or
- to prevent the offender from committing further offences.

(HO/Probation Service Division, 1992)

Effective supervision will also entail establishing a professional relationship in which to advise, assist and befriend the offender with the aim of:

- securing the offender's co-operation and compliance with the probation order and enforcing its terms;
- challenging the offender to accept responsibility for his or her crime and its consequences;
- helping the offender to resolve personal difficulties linked with offending and to acquire new skills; and
- motivating and assisting the offender to become a responsible and law-abiding member of the community.

(HO/Probation Service Division, 1992)

Where the order includes a condition of psychiatric treatment, there will be the added dimension of working with and alongside the psychiatric services. However, if the offender is receiving treatment as an in-patient, direct supervision is not required although the officer retains the responsibility for revocation or amendment of the order. If treatment is on an out-patient basis, supervision should be conducted in the normal manner but liaising closely with those providing the treatment.

It is this latter requirement that seems to cause most problems with such orders. Although the order has the potential for providing a focal point between social work, law and medicine there is often confusion between all parties involved. A study by Lewis (1980) of all the probation orders in force in Nottinghamshire in 1978 showed that the offenders were unsure of what was on offer; the probation officers had expectations of the doctors that were too high and the doctors had little appreciation of the probation officers' contribution. Unfortunately, the problems caused by lack of co-operation appear to have continued to this day. Mr G. Smith, Chief Probation Officer for the Inner London Probation Service, speaking at the 20th Cropwood Conference in 1990, described the 'separate track' working of the order. He commented on the offenders' not infrequent breakdown because they had stopped taking their medication and of the side-effects of drugs interfering with initiative and spontaneity. He also regretted that the essential degree of professional closeness necessary to deal with this problem had not been fully grasped by either service (Smith, 1993).

And yet this does not have to be the case. Smith emphasizes that the probation service can succeed only if there is a meaningful liaison between itself and psychiatry, and he goes on to quote an example of The Netherlands, where most probation teams have the regular support of their own consultant psychiatrist. In the UK, the Hertfordshire Panel Scheme referred to above seems to have made the management of such an order a truly multidisciplinary affair, although the probation officer retains responsibility as the supervising officer.

In order to make these probation orders work, proper care must be taken in the selection of potential probationers. They need to be able to benefit from treatment in the community, be prepared to respect the authority of the order and not pose a risk to the public. At the outset of the order, a clear supervision plan needs to be made which is agreed by and shared with the offender. The professionals involved, particularly the probation officer and psychiatrist, should clarify their intentions and respective roles with each other. Above all, they should meet face to face on a regular basis to ensure coordination is maintained. Only if such orders are seen to be managed effectively will courts follow recommendations 11.17 of the Reed Report that 'the possible use of probation orders with a condition of psychiatric treatment should be considered more frequently' (D of H/HO, 1992).

SUPERVISION AND TREATMENT ORDER UNDER THE CRIMINAL PROCEDURE (INSANITY AND UNFITNESS TO PLEAD) ACT 1991

This Act, which became effective on 1 January 1992, introduced a new community disposal option: the Supervision and Treatment Order. The Act itself is used in cases where the accused person has been found unfit to be tried and enables a trial of the facts to be carried out. Where the accused is found to have done the act or made the omission charged against him or is found not guilty by reason of insanity, the court may choose to impose a Supervision and Treatment Order. Such an order would normally be made when the person requires and may be susceptible to treatment but whose psychiatric condition does not warrant an admission to hospital or the making of a Guardianship Order.

Additionally, such an order cannot be made unless the supervising officer named in the order is willing to undertake the supervision and arangements have been made for the treatment intended, to be specified in the order. The order will require the accused to be under the supervision of a social worker or probation officer for a specified period of up to two years. In reality the social supervision will probably be provided by social workers perhaps attached to the same hospital or clinical team as the doctor carrying out the treatment. This would ensure consistency and access to facilities available for the support of the mentally disordered person. It may be, however, that in some cases probation supervision would be preferable, particularly if the person is already known to the probation service.

The order is not considered to be a punitive measure. It is modelled on the Probation Order with a Condition of Psychiatric Treatment and is for use in cases where the court is satisfied that release into the community will not pose an unacceptable risk to the safety of the public. The subject of the order therefore will probably be able to look after himself in his own home and will have been charged with a relatively minor offence. The aim is to ensure that such persons receive medical treatment either as an in-patient for a short period or as an out-patient, and receive social support to help them keep within the law.

The agency responsible for discharging the order will have a supporting role. The duties to be undertaken will depend on the individual circumstances of each case. As with the probation order with special conditions described above, the supervising officer will be expected to liaise, as appropriate, with the medical and nursing services, and take any steps necessary to help the person cope in the community. Such steps might include finding suitable accommodation, ensuring that the person is kept reasonably occupied and dealing with any day-to-day problems that might arise.

Unlike the probation order, the supervision and treatment order is not dependent on the person's willingness to accept it. Indeed, because of his mental condition he is unlikely to be able to give meaningful consent. However, if at any time he refuses to co-operate with his supervision or treatment, the court has no power to enforce the order or otherwise intervene in cases of non-compliance. If it is felt that the supervisee is in need of treatment against his will, then the appropriate action should be taken under the Mental Health Act 1983. The supervisor may report to the court in writing at any time to amend or revoke the order if it is considered in the interests of the health and welfare of the supervised person.

GUARDIANSHIP ORDERS

Guardianship was originally introduced into legislation at the behest of the eugenics movement as a way of controlling the sexual behaviour of mentally handicapped people. Its use has changed considerably over time and is now seen as a supportive measure. Current legislation allows a guardianship order to be made in cases where the criteria for the making of a hospital order apply but that the mental disorder is of a nature and degree that warrants reception into guardianship. The making of such an order enables the guardian, who may be the local authority or other responsible person, to:

1. decide where the patient shall live;
2. require attendance at centres for treatment, occupation

education or training (although not to require the person
to have treatment when they get there);

3. require access to the patient to be given to the medical practitioner or approved social worker or other persons
specified by the guardian to any place where the patient
is residing.

Such orders can be made for 'civil' patients under Section 7,
Mental Health Act 1983 and for mentally disordered offenders
under Section 37, Mental Health Act 1983 or under the
Criminal Proceedings (Insanity and Unfitness to Plead) Act
1991. Although the Mental Health Act 1983 modified the power
of the guardian from previous legislation, the guardianship
order remains essentially a device to exercise social control in
the community. The Code of Practice for the Mental Health
Act 1983 (D of H/Welsh Office, 1993) defines the purpose of
guardianship as follows:

> The purpose of guardianship is to enable patients to receive
> community care where it cannot be provided without the
> use of compulsory powers. It enables the establishment of
> an authoritative framework for workimg with a patient with
> a minimum of constraint to achieve as independent a life
> a possible within the community. Where it is used it
> must be part of the patient's overall care and treatment
> plan.

It further states that 'Guardianship orders may be particularly
suitable in helping to meet the needs of mentally impaired
offenders who could benefit from occupation, training and
education in the community.'

However, experience has shown that there has been a
downturn in its use for people suffering from mental impairment and severe mental impairment since 1983 with a small
increase in its use for people with mental illness (Hughes,
1990/91). This is probably due to the rather tight definition of
mental impairment and the more undefined definition of
mental illness. Even with the slight increase in the use of guardianship for people with mental illness, its use remains small
particularly for its application through the Courts. Indeed,
research by Millington (1989) showed that guardianship orders
are the least used provision in the criminal code.

There are a number of reasons why this is so. Most guardianship orders are made in favour of the local authority as opposed to any other appropriate person. Nevertheless, local authorities are reluctant to take on such responsibilities and, in the area of offender patients, there is the added caution of not wishing to enter an area of social control that is unfamiliar to them. The acceptance of an order obliges the local authority to commit resources to the individual in terms of residential care, daycare provision and community support. Many authorities would take the view that they are being financially unfairly burdened for an area of work that is not necessarily within their remit. If the offender received a prison sentence, the Home Office would bear the cost; if a hospital order was made, the health authority would meet the bill. With the wider responsibility of the NHS and Community Care Act 1990 upon them, local authorities are even less inclined to welcome mentally disordered offenders with open arms.

In any event, before the court can make a guardianship order it has to be satisfied that the local authority is willing to act as guardian. The reality is that local authorities have no liking for them and cannot be forced to accept them. Interestingly, Section 27 of the Criminal Justice Act 1991 extends Section 39 of the Mental Health Act 1983 to enable a social services department to be required to attend court to explain whether it is willing to accept an offender into guardianship and to give such information as it reasonably can about how it could be expected to exercise its powers.

In cases where such orders are made, their success depends largely upon the co-operation of the person subject to guardianship. There must be a willingness on the part of both parties to work together within the terms of the authority vested in the guardian by the Act. Although, for instance, the guardian can require the person to live at a specified place, there is no legal authority to detain him there physically against his will. Similarly, while the patient can be required to attend at specified places for medical treatment, occupation or training, force cannot be used to secure such attendance. Nor can medical treatment be given without the patient's consent. As with all forms of work with this group, much will depend on the establishment of a supportive and trusting relationship with a clear understanding of each others' responsibilities and mutually agreed goals. Moreover, a multidisciplinary approach using a comprehensive care plan will ensure clear direction and support for the worker.

In the event of non-compliance, however, there is no provision to return the offender to court. If he is in need of treatment he may have to be admitted to hospital on a compulsory basis under the Mental Health Act 1983. If he re-offends he will have to be brought before the court and dealt with afresh. On balance, therefore, the use of a guardianship order for the mentally disordered offender may be more suitable for the inadequate recidivist as the provision of accommodation, occupation, training and medical treatment may keep him out of prison.

However, from the court's point of view local authorities are not associated with criminal responsibilities and the use of the probation service tends to be the preferred option. Where community supervision with an option treatment is thought to be the most appropriate disposal option, the court may prefer to use a probation order with a condition of psychiatric treatment.

THE CARE PROGRAMME APPROACH

Introduced in April 1991 the Care Programme Approach (CPA) requires District Health Authorities with Social Services collaboration to ensure that all patients accepted by specialist mental health services have a care plan and named key worker in place to minimize the possibility of individuals with severe mental illness losing contact with those services (D of H, 1990).

The essential elements of a CPA are systematic assessment, a care plan, the allocation of a key worker and regular review. The task of the key worker is to keep in close contact with the patient, monitor the agreed programme of care and take immediate action in the event of difficulties in providing that care. In order to work effectively, the CPA required close inter-disciplinary and inter-personal working so that a co-ordinated response can be made to individual needs.

Although a health-led procedure, the key worker may be from any agency or profession, including representatives from organized voluntary bodies. Where mentally disordered offenders are included in the procedcures, the CPA meetings should include representatives from the criminal justice agencies. Indeed, mentally disordered offenders are prime candidates for CPAs because they are a particularly vulnerable group. It is important therefore that effective links are formed between local agencies and supra-district services such as special hospitals and medium secure units so that they can work jointly with them in planning effective after-care arrangements on discharge. Similarly, NACRO makes proposals for extending the CPA to include prisoners identified as being mentally ill, so that no such prisoners are released without appropriate plans and arrangements for their care in the community (NACRO/Mental Health Advisory Committee, 1993).

As with all interventions, it is good practice and more likely to work if the patient is fully involved in the process. All patients should be invited to the CPA assessment meeting and subsequent reviews and be involved in the planning of care and support systems. This should also include relatives or carers as appropriate. If patients are too confused to contribute to their assessment reviews, then decisions must be made for them by members of the multidisciplinary team and carers/relatives/advocates. Discontinuance of the care programme should occur when the patient is seen as no longer vulnerable although it may be prudent to maintain contact as long as is considered necessary.

SUPERVISION REGISTERS

Supervision Registers were introduced on 1 April 1994 and required NHS Provider Units to set up registers that identify and provide information on patients who:

1. are over 16 years of age; and
2. have a diagnosis of mental illness (including personality disorder of psychopathic disorders who are receiving treatment from a specialist psychiatric service); and
3. are known to be at significant risk or potentially significant risk to suicide, serious violence to others or severe self-neglect (NHS Management Executive, 1994).

The aim of the register is to ensure that people with a severe mental illness, and who are significantly at risk, receive appropriate and effective care in the community. Although there was strong support for such measures from some quarters, notably the Report of the Inquiry into the Care and Treatment of Christopher Clunis (Ritchie *et al.*, 1994), it also raised issues of civil liberties. Unlike the application of the Mental Health Act 1983 which gives patients access to a tribunal system, no such measures are available in applying the register. It is very important therefore that community-based workers involved in the process ensure that the patient has every opportunity to be involved in the discussion about registration.

Consideration for inclusion on the register should not be done in isolation and should form part of the Care Programme Approach assessment and review meetings. Although the decision for inclusion rests with the consultant psychiatrist responsible for the patient's care, there should be consultation with others involved with the patient. The key workers should ensure that patients and, where they wish, an advocate, relative, friend or carer, have an opportunity to state their views through attendance at the Care Programme Approach meeting or through discussion with the relevant clinicians and key worker.

Having been put on the register patients should be informed orally and in writing that they have been put on the register, why they have been put on it, how the information will be used, to whom it will be disclosed and the mechanism for review.

The register should provide a point of reference for relevant and authorized health and social services staff to enquire whether individuals under the Care Programme are at risk. It also identifies those patients who should receive the highest priority for care and active follow-up. What it does not do, however, is generate extra resources. Nevrtheless, workers with such patients on their caseloads need to be particularly diligent in their care and supervision and provide a rapid response to their needs in times of crisis.

Removal from the register may be considered at the request of any agency of professional involved in the patient's care or at the request of the patient himself. Consideration for removal should also be considered at every Care Programme Approach review meeting, the final decision again resting with the consultant psychiatrist in consultation with the relevant staff involved.

SUMMARY

It is likely that most professionals in the mental health and criminal justice systems have a number of invisible or unrecognized mentally disordered offenders on their caseload. There will be offenders who have an unrecognized and untreated mental illness and people with mental illness who are potential or 'uncharged' offenders. It is argued that if they can be recognized at the primary stage, then more appropriate services can be utilized early in their deviant or psychiatric careers. However, in doing so there is always the danger of further stigmatizing of the client and reinforcing the public's misconceptions about people with mental disorders automatically being associated with crime. Nevertheless, on occasion it may be in the public and client's interest to pursue such a course, particularly for those clients who are aggressive and threatening. On balance, there is probably a greater risk from neglecting such features than in appropriately intervening with authoritarian measures.

For those clients already identified as mentally disordered offenders, there are a number of government directives, policies and legislative measures which help form the appropriate care and supervision framework in the community. These range through diversion from custody at the police station, to the targeting of vulnerable individuals, to specific court orders to oversee the mentally disordered offender in order to avoid the necessity for institutional care.

REFERENCES

Barker, R.L. and Branson, D.H. (1993) *Forensic Social Work: Legal Aspects of Professional Practice*, The Howarth Press, New York.

Bowden, P. (1978) Men remanded into custody for medical reports: the selection for treatment. *British Journal of Psychiatry*, **132**, 320–31.

Cohen, J. and Fisher, M. (1987) Recognition of mental health problems by doctors and social workers. *Practice*, **1**(3), 225–40.

Department of Health (1990) *Care Programme Approach (CPA) for People with a Mental Illness Referred to the Specialist Psychiatric Services*, HC (90) 23, LASSL (90) 11, Department of Health, London.

Department of Health (1993) *The Health of the Nation Key Area Handbook: Mental Illness*, HMSO, London.

Department of Health and Home Office (1992) *Review of Health and Social Services for Mentally Disordered Offenders and Others Requiring*

Similar Services. Final Summary Report Cmnd 2088, HMSO, London.

Department of Health and Welsh Office (1993) *Code of Practice Mental Health Act 1983*, Revised edn. HMSO, London.

Hedderman, C. (1993) *Panel Assessment Schemes for Mentally Disordered Offenders*, Research and Unit Planning Paper No. 76, Home Office, London.

Hodgins, S. (ed.) (1993) *Mental Disorder and Crime*, Sage, London.

Home Office (1990) *Provision for Mentally Disordered Offenders*, Home Office Circular No. 66/90, Home Office, London.

Home Office (1991) *Police and Criminal Evidence Act 1984 (section 66) Codes of Practice*, revised edn, HMSO, London.

Home Office (1993) *Mentally Disordered Offenders: Draft Circular on Diversion*, 28 June, Home Office, London.

Home Office Probation Service Division (1992) *National Standards for the Supervision of Offenders in the Community*, HMSO, London.

Home Office and Department of Health (1993) *Examples of Good Practice and information about diversion Initiatives*, HMSO, London.

Hughes, G. (1990/91) Trends in guardianship usage following the Mental Health Act 1983. *Health Trends*, Vol. 22, No. 4, 145–7.

Joseph, P.L. and Potter, M. (1990) Mentally disordered homeless offenders – diversion from custody. *Health Trends*, Vol. 2, No. 2, 51–3.

Lewis, P. (1980) *Psychiatric Probation Orders: Roles and Expectations of Probation Officers and Psychiatrists*, Institute of Criminology, University of Cambridge, Cambridge.

Major, J. (1991) What can a magistrate do? in *The Mentally Disordered Offender* (eds. K. Herbert and J. Gunn) Butterworth-Heinemann, Oxford, pp. 46–64.

Millington, S. (1989) Guardianship and the Mental Health Act 1983. Social Work Monographs, University of East Anglia, Norwich.

NACRO Mental Health Advisory Committee (1993) *Community Care and Mentally Disturbed Offenders*, Policy Paper 1, NACRO, London.

NHS Management Executive (1994) *Introduction of Supervision Registers for Mentally Ill People from 1 April 1994*, Health Service Guidelines HSG (94)5, NHS, London.

National Practitioners Group (1993) *Newsletter*, 2nd edn., July, National Practitioners Group, Warley.

North Humberside MIND (1993) *Diversion from Custody Project: Briefing Paper*, North Humberside MIND, Hull.

Onyett, S. (1992) *Case Management in Mental Health*, Chapman & Hall, London.

Patmore, C. and Weaver, T. (1992) Improving community services for serious mental disorders. *Journal of Mental Health*, 1, 107–15.

Ritchie, J.H., Dick, D. and Lingham, R. (1994) *The Report of the Inquiry into the Care and Treatment of Christopher Clunis*, presented to the Chairman of North East Thames and South East Thames Regional Health Authorities, HMSO, London.

Shepherd, G. (1993) Case management, in *The Mentally Disordered Offender in an Era of Community Care: New Directions in Provision*, (eds W. Watson and A. Grounds), Cambridge University Press, Cambridge, pp. 166–76.

Smith, G.W. (1993) A view from the probation service, in *The Mentally Disordered Offender In An Era of Community Care: New Directions In Provision*, (eds W. Watson and A. Grounds), Cambridge University Press, Cambridge, pp. 118–26.

Sone, K. (1990) At the mercy of the law. *Community Care*, 18 October, 28–30.

Steadman, H.J. and Cocozza, J.J. (1974) *Careers of the Criminally Insane*, Lexington Books, Lexington.

Watson, W. (1993) Future directions for research, in *The Mentally Disordered Offender in an Era of Community Care: New Directions in Provision*, (eds W. Watson and A. Grounds), Cambridge University Press, Cambridge, pp. 191–200.

6

Supervision of patients subject to special restrictions

WORK WITHIN THE HOSPITAL SETTING

Forensic social work as a specialism is a relatively new development. Although there have been social work teams located in psychiatric hospitals for many years, their support for mentally disordered offenders has been minimal, if only because conventional psychiatric hospitals have for some considerable time gradually retreated from providing a service to these patients. Most of the expertise, therefore, has been concentrated in the special hospitals of Ashworth, Rampton and Broadmoor in England and Carstairs in Scotland. It is only very recently that the specialism has been developed further with the emergence of the Regional Secure Units and Court Diversion Schemes.

Even so, there are still only a relatively few workers dedicated entirely to work with this client group, and it was not until the publication of the Aarvold Report in 1973 (HO/DHSS, 1973) that social work along with other professions was officially recognized as having a valid voice in the recommendations for discharge of special hospital patients. The report was commissioned by the government following the discharge from Broadmoor Hospital in February 1971 of Graham Young who was subsequently convicted of murder and other grave offences committed by poisoning, in the period between his leaving hospital and his arrest in November 1971.

Consequently, the Aarvold Committee was asked to advise 'whether the procedures now approved for the discharge and supervision of patients subject to special restrictions under Section 65 of the Mental Health Act 1959, are satisfactory or whether there are further changes within the existing law, which should be made'. In its deliberations the committee noted the value of multidisciplinary case conferences and expressed the hope that they would become common practice. It did realize however, that 'it may be some time before the staff situation at some hospitals makes this possible'. Indeed, in 1973 the social work influence in the special hospital system was minimal. At Broadmoor Hospital, for instance, the first qualified social worker was not employed until 1969. Before then the hospital had been served by a few unqualified welfare officers and the recommendations of the Aarvold Committee provided a much-needed boost to the social work input to such institutions. Particularly relevant was the recommendation: 'That wherever possible the recommendation of a responsible medical officer for the discharge of a restricted patient from hospital, or for transfer from a secure hospital to one in the National Health Service, should be supported by the recorded views of other professional personnel, such as nursing, occupational, psychological and social work staff, with knowledge of and responsibility for the patient, including his rehabilitation.' Consequently, in the 20 years since the Aarvold Report, special hospital social workers have grown from humble beginnings as minor officials with little influence to a group of specialist workers with improved status and an important part to play in the overall care, treatment and rehabilitation of patients. Nevertheless, such developments have not been easy, and an early account by Vaughan (1979) gives an insight into the difficulties of establishing a social work presence in such a closed institution.

Even today social work does not always sit easily within the special hospital system. Interestingly, social work does not have direct representation on the hospital management committees and is subsumed under the Rehabilitation Directorates. Moreover, the enquiry into Ashworth Special Hospital in 1992 said that social workers were obliged to play a marginal role in patient care and 'were outside the mainstream of patient-care decisions'. It went further in criticizing the service for being professionally isolated from social work colleagues in related fields' (Marchant, 1993).

Without doubt, special hospitals are difficult settings in which to work. With the best will in the world it is difficult for workers themselves to remain unaffected by the insidious effects of institutionalization. Unlike other social workers, they are employed by the Special Hospitals Service Authority and are also geographically separated from their professional colleagues. It is difficult to retain the critical independence needed for their role and easy to be seduced by the mores of the system. Accordingly, special hospital social workers are a small, self supporting group of workers whose activities are often tempered by the culture of the host institutions.

Social workers based in Regional Secure Units share some of these difficulties but in the main have much more freedom and independence. Employed by the local authorities they are more closely linked into mainstream social work and the local community.

Against this backdrop, social work with the hospital order patients subject to special restrictions is undertaken while the latter remains an in-patient. The actual role of the social worker in such settings can be nearly divided into three distinct areas related to admission, throughcare and discharge/transfer.

Admission

The largest single group of patients admitted to the special hospitals are those subject to a Hospital Order under Section 37 of the Mental Health Act 1983 and in most cases also attracting a restriction order without limit of time under Section 41. About 10% are transferred from prison under Section 47 with a restriction direction usually added by the Home Secretary. A mere handful are admitted each year under Section 5 of the Criminal Procedure (Insanity and Unfitness to Plead) Act 1991. A further 20% of special hospital patients are on long-term civil commitment orders following their transfer from an NHS hospital.

Despite what may have been a prolonged period of investigation and treatment in other settings, admission to a forensic unit triggers a fresh appraisal of the situation in which the social worker has an important part to play. During the initial the patient to establish a rapport, ascertain the extent of family links, deal with practical issues, liaise with outside agencies, etc. However, perhaps the most useful role will be in contributing to the multidisciplinary assessment process by gathering important background information from relatives and other agencies.

Most agencies will already be known to a number of other agencies. They will often have experienced being in the care of the local authority as children, have been known to the probation service because of previous offences or will have had contact with local authority social workers while in-patients at local psychiatric hospitals. Collating such information even within one agency is often a mammoth task, one which is often overlooked by community social workers and probation officers. However, a comprehensive account of the involvement of other community agencies helps build up a valuable portrait of the patient's psychiatric and criminal career. Only if a full and detailed account of the patient's history is made available to the multidisciplinary team can some understanding be gained of the patient's behaviour and how his illness has developed.

A rich source of such information is the patient's family. However, many months will have usually elapsed between the offence and the final admission to hospital and a family visit shortly afterwards needs to be handled sensitively. For many families such a visit will simply re-open old wounds and bring them face-to-face with their trauma once more. Consider the following case example:

Case study

Brian H., a 27-year-old single man, was admitted to a special hospital after stabbing his mother to death in a frenzied attack during a psychotic phase of his schizophrenic illness. The social worker from the hospital arranged to see Brian's father at the family home shortly after admission. Although Brian's father did his best to help the social worker with background information, the interview had to be terminated when Brian's father became hostile and finally broke down. It became evident during the interview that the offence had been committed in the very room where the interview was being conducted and had been witnessed by Brian's father. After the event, Brian's

> father had been offered no counselling or support and had
> never had an opportunity to talk about the incident to anybody.
> The social worker's visit was the first time since the offence
> that Brian's father had an opportunity of sharing his feelings
> about the horrific event that had befallen his family.

This is clearly a fruitful area of work for the social worker. While not all initial visits are as traumatic as the example above, the social worker is often faced with unresolvedfamily feelings about the offence and the patient. Unfortunately, local agencies tend not to involve themselves in such matters and families are often left to cope unaided. Sensitive, careful preparation for such visits is needed to avoid any unnecessary distress.

On other occasions it may be difficult to engage relations at all, as prolonged, disruptive behaviour of the patient prior to admission may have eroded much of the goodwill that previously existed. Contact with the family is without doubt a crucial element of the social work task and the initial visit may well influence the family's subsequent contact with the hospital and the patient. Finally, it should be remembered that some patients are detained in special hospitals because they *have* got relatives outside. Because of their own disordered behaviour the visits of some relatives prove to be detrimental to patients. Others who may have been assaulted by the patient in a setting of delusional jealousy may do better by severing their relationship altogether if the patient is ever to have the opportunity of a risk-free discharge.

Throughcare

Unlike those detained in other custodial institutions such as prison, who have a definite release date, those patients detained in hospital under Section 37 of the Mental Health Act 1983 face an indeterminate period of incarceration with an average length of stay of about eight years in the special hospitals. Some are obviously detained for much longer periods; the record is held by a William Giles who died in Broadmoor at the age of 87, having being detained for 76 years. The regional secure units on the other hand are intended to take patients who require treatment in the short term not usually exceeding 18 months to two years.

With such a prolonged length of stay it is easy for the therapeutic thrust to be overtaken by the insidious effects of institutionalization. To compound matters the special hospitals have traditionally served a national catchment area and although these have now been regionalized there are still many patients with families scattered all over the country. Maintaining meaningful contact over an indefinite period of time can be difficult if not daunting. A survey of 132 Long-stay Broadmoor patients showed that a large number were neglected by their families and also that many were socially isolated before their admission (Vaughan, 1980).

In view of the potential for patients to become isolated and lose contact with the outside world, an active throughcare programme is vital. If the main function of social work in such settings is linked to the prime aim of the hospital, i.e. the discharge and transfer of its patients, then it has an important role in helping to provide conditions that facilitate this aim. One of the social worker's activities, therefore, must be an attempt to preserve social contact with the outside world, particularly in relation to families. This would seem essential if many patients are not to find themselves without any meaningful support from relatives after discharge.

The social worker needs to be active in identifying those patients who are most isolated in an effort to promote some or more contact with the outside world. Motivational groups for chronic institutionalized patients could be encouraged along with a wider use of remedial education and literacy classes to activate patients in letter-writing. Relatives should not be left for long periods of time without any official contact with the hospital, as this is likely to lead to resentment when they are eventually asked to take a more active interest on discharge. Regular feedback to relatives could possibly do much to forestall diminishing interest over the years and might help maintain a feeling of commitment to the patient.

Unfortunately, such activities are bound to be limited given the caseloads of special hospital social workers who are unlikely to have less than 50 patients on their caseloads. With families scattered all over the country, frequent contact is simply not possible for all. At Broadmoor, for instance, a performance target is for one family visit per year (Personal Communication with Social Work Department, 1993).

One way of extending such contact is to engage probation officers and local authority social workers in the task. Probation offcers have a tradition of throughcare for their charges, and where this is maintained it can prove to be a great asset. Local authority social workers, however, are much less inclined to maintain contact particularly where distances are great.

In addition to the above are the normal range of duties social workers carry out in ordinary psychiatric hospitals depending on their particular interests, skills and patient needs. However, the biggest investment in time and effort is likely to be expended on transfer/discharge arrangements.

Transfer/discharge

Patients subject to special restrictions who are detained in special hospitals may be discharged directly into the community, although transfer to a Regional Secure Unit or local psychiatric hospital is more common. When a discharge or transfer is thought appropriate by the responsible medical officer, a recommendation, which should be supported by members of the multidisciplinary team, including the social worker, is made to the Home Secretary. In considering his response the Home Secretary will take into account whether there is an adequate understanding of how the patient came to commit the offence that led to his detention in hospital, evidence that a change has taken place while in hospital so that he is unlikely to commit further serious offences and whether he has a sensible and realistic view of his future life in the community.

In addition to the above an intermediary stage was introduced following the Aarvold Report (HO/DHSS, 1973) for the small proportion of restricted patients in whose case the risk of serious re-offending was particularly difficult to predict. An advisory board was established to consider the transfer/ discharge recommendations before the Home Secretary gave his consent to them. There are no criteria to determine which cases are referred to the Board and it is left to the judgement of the responsible medical officer or Home Secretary to decide on appropriate cases. The number of proposals referred to the Board remain steady at around 50 per year (Baxter, 1991).

Notwithstanding the above, the restricted patient also has access, at periodic intervals, to the Mental Health Act Review Tribunal. The Tribunal has the power to direct a conditional discharge if satisfied that one of two statutory criteria are met:

1. the patient is not suffering from a form of mental disorder which makes it inappropriate for him to be liable to be maintained in hospital for medical treatment; or
2. that it is not necessary for the health or safety of the patient or for the protection of other persons that he should receive such treatment.

The only exception is for prisoners who have been transferred to hospital and are subject to restriction directions under Section 49. Such patients would not be discharged but would return to prison to complete their sentence.

Social workers from inside and outside the hospital setting will be required to conduct the necessary investigations and submit a social report for each Tribunal sitting. This is no small undertaking, given that there is an MHRT hearing approximately every working day in each special hospital (Hamilton, 1990).

Despite these mechanisms, the process of moving a patient out of the special hospital system tends to be slow and tortuous. Although an MHRT might agree to the discharge of a restricted patient, it is common for the actual discharge date to be deferred until the appropriate community support systems are in place. Where a recommendation for transfer or discharge is made to the Home Secretary, there may be lengthy delays before it is even considered, particularly if the case first has to be put before the Aarvold Board. When a final agreement is reached, further delays are usually experienced in finding a local hospital willing to accept the patient. Such delays can sometimes be very lengthy. Hamilton quotes an example in 1986 of 32 patients who had been waiting more than three years, including five patients who had been waiting more than six years for transfer (Hamilton, 1990). Such delays led the Mental Health Act Commission to make a number of recommendations to reduce the waiting time for transfer and discharge and thus alleviate some of the distress and frustration felt by the patients who are affected (Mental Health Act Commission, 1987).

Social workers among other staff often need to spend much time sustaining patients who have to wait months and even years beyond their expected leaving date. A further area of activity for the social worker at this time is in rehabilitation programmes designed to prepare patients to face the outside world once more. Escorted leave and preparatory visits to prospective hostels are needed to 'test out' patients in the real world, although the demand on staff time is such that these excursions are not numerous enough. Of particular difficulty is planning a rehabilitation programme that will fit in with a constantly extended leaving date due to the difficulties mentioned above. Unlike social work in prison where working with inmates towards a definite release date is possible, social work in special hospitals is problematic given a constantly deferred leaving date (Vaughan and Fortt, 1983).

During this time, further contact needs to be made with the family to prepare them for the impending move. Hopefully, contact would have been maintained during the earlier years as research has shown that the continued interest and support of family members for the mentally disordered offender does have a favourable influence on the patient's prospects of leaving the hospital (Steadman and Cocozza, 1974; Dell, 1980). Nevertheless, some relatives become alarmed and resentful when the patient reaches the stage of transfer or discharge. Some families will have drifted away from the patient and will have regrouped without him. Any approach that is made, especially in relation to transfer or discharge, may re-open old wounds and arouse fear and resentment. The result is not uncommonly a retreat by some relatives from active involvement in the patient's future.

In cases of direct discharge into the community it is usually left to the social worker to make arrangements to secure appropriate accommodation. Occasionally, a patient may return to the family home but it is more usual for him to be discharged into a supervised hostel where his rehabilitation can be continued. Finding such accommodation, however, is not easy. The starting point is to look for accommodation in the patient's home area but often his admission offence and/or previous disturbed behaviour in the community may have alienated the local community against him. Furthermore, hostel staff are very wary of patients who might have committed the most horrendous admission offence and feel that they do not have the skills and resources to take them on.

Forensic social workers are exposed to such patients every day and are sometimes seduced into accepting appalling offences as 'normal'. It is easy to forget the feelings of revulsion and fear that the public has for some categories of mentally disordered offender. The following case is an example of such a situation:

Case study

John, a 42-year-old butcher, lived with his wife and five children in a small country village. He developed a severe endogenous depressive illness during which he became psychotic. At this time he believed that the world was wicked and sinful and was not a fit place in which he and his family should live. Accordingly one night when they were all asleep he strangled his wife in her bed and then cut the throats of each of his five daughters. He subsequently made a failed suicide attempt and was eventually admitted to a special hospital.

On admission he quickly responded to treatment and when he realized the full horror of what had happened, he developed a severe reactive depressive illness. Nevertheless, after about two years as an in-patient he was thought to be stable enough to be considered for discharge. On interview the hospital social worker found John to be a very amenable man and quickly established a good relationship with him, giving no thought to the magnitude of the offence as it was no more horrific than those of many other patients he had worked with.

The social worker was subsequently surprised and disappointed at the repeated rebuffs from hostel staff when he made overtures to them for a placement. Moreover, the local community petitioned their MP and the Queen against John returning to the neighbourhood once they discovered a discharge was being planned.

The social worker thought these reactions unreasonable until reminded in supervision that his was the unreasonable reaction and the community's reaction was understandable.

However, even less dramatic cases can be equally hard to place. Under Section 117 of the Mental Health Act 1983 social services departments have a duty to provide appropriate after-care for previously detained patients. Unfortunately, social services departments rarely have such facilities or indeed the funding for residential care. Mental health hostels are usually over-subscribed and reluctant to take mentally disordered offenders either because of their apprehension or simply not having adequate supervisory cover. In any event, many hostels offer only short-term placements which are not always suitable for the longer-term rehabilitation needs of the more disabled offender.

With the growth of the independent sector since the implementation of the NHS and Community Care Act 1990 it may be that this niche in the market will be filled. Nevertheless, there will still be difficulties in securing adequate funding from hard-pressed local authorities.

The final phase of the in-patient social work task will be to facilitate the introduction and handover to a social supervisor from the community whose task it will be to supervise the subsequent discharge arrangements.

SUPERVISION IN THE COMMUNITY

There are currently about 1700 restricted patients detained in mental hospitals of whom about 1100 are to be found in the special hospitals. At any one time there are about 600–700 conditionally discharged patients under active supervision in the community. With such low numbers spread all over the country, the experience of supervising an ex-special hospital patient comes relatively rarely to individual social workers and probation officers. It is therefore difficult for individual workers to develop a body of knowledge and gain experience for this demanding task.

For most long-term psychiatric patients, rehabilitation and resettlement into the community after many years of hospital care are difficult enough. For the mentally disordered offender who will have been incarcerated in a top security institution for an average of more than eight years (Hamilton, 1990) such difficulties will be compounded enormously. Having lost contact with the outside world for many years, he will face an alien and often hostile world on discharge. The public is not renowned for its sympathy for and understanding of the mentally ill nor its willingness to offer support to those with a criminal background. The mentally disordered offender suffers the dual stigma of mental illness and criminality and is often considered both 'mad' and 'bad'. Moreover, the restricted patient is likely to have committed a particularly serious and/or bizarre offence which will make his acceptance into the community especially difficult. It is against this background that a social worker or probation officer accepts the role of a social supervisor and at the same time has to face his own anxieties and fears.

Although a small proportion of restricted patients are discharged direct from special hospital into the community, the more usual route is through an intermediate stage of transfer to a local psychiatric hospital or Regional Secure Unit. From here the patient will receive further rehabilitation, a reintroduction to community life, trial leave and finally discharge, usually to a form of supervised accommodation. However, whatever the route the same rigorous rules and conditions will govern his discharge.

All conditionally discharged restricted patients are subject to strict conditions relating to their after-care in the community. These are invariably:

1. residence at a stated address;
2. supervision by a local authority social worker or a probation officer; and
3. psychiatric supervision.

Occasionally additional conditions may be stipulated, such as not being within a certain radius of a particular location. Guidelines are also issued for social supervisors (HO/DHSS, 1987a), supervising psychiatrists (HO/DHSS, 1987b) and hospitals (HO/DHSS, 1987c) which fully explain the process, preparation and after-care requirements.

Preparation for supervision

During the patient's stay in hospital, the hospital social work department will have maintained links with outside individuals and agencies who may be able to offer support to the patient after discharge. Although there are difficulties of distance and competing demands on services, such efforts will be rewarded by a greater commitment to the patient on leaving hospital. As part of their planning the multidisciplinary team should have a clear idea of the arrangements in the community which will best suit the patient, including the agency most likely to provide the best supervision and support.

Since the Mental Health Act 1959 both social workers and probation officers have been undertaking this task. Their current statutory obligations are spelt out under the general duties expressed in Section 117 of the Mental Health Act 1983 and under the probation rules. Both agencies have the skills and experience in providing such care and in working with the relevant services, and it is usually possible to identify a suitable social supervisor within them. Very occasionally, however, another individual such as a community psychiatric nurse may be the best choice in a particular case and would be considered by the Home Office (HO/DHSS, 1987c).

The factors determining the choice of supervising agency are sometimes self-evident. For example, one agency may have been supervising the patient before admission, maintained throughcare contact and already have a good relationship with him. If plans are being made for the patient to be discharged to a particular hostel it may be that one or other of the agencies is already involved in its management. In practice, where the patient has a clearly defined mental illness with an ongoing need for treatment and monitoring of his mental state, a specialist mental health social worker is the likely choice. On the other hand Mace (1991) quotes the Home Secretary as saying that 'the probation service would be expected to be the agency nominated to supervise discharged special hospital patients whose criminal offences carried a life sentence penalty where they had not been diagnosed as mentally ill and in need of hospital treatment.'

Where a choice is clearcut the hospital social work department should approach the appropriate Director of Social Services or the Chief Probation Officer, giving the relevant information about the patient and the discharge plans, with a request for a suitable supervising officer to be nominated. Where such a clear choice is not possible, both agencies should be invited to send a representative to a predischarge case conference where the choice of agency can be determined.

Once a social supervisor has been nominated he should be involved as early as practicable in the planning and preparation for the patient's discharge. It is recommended in the guidelines that a minimum of two visits to the hospital be made by the social supervisor and that he should be involved in at least one case conference. If involved early enough, the social supervisor can sometimes be usefully involved in the preparation of community links, accommodation, family support, etc. In any event, the discharging hospital should ensure that a comprehensive set of information is made available prior to discharge. As a minimum the package should consist of the following:

1. a pen-picture of the patient, including his diagnosis and current mental state;
2. admission, social and medical history;
3. summary of progress in hospital;
4. present medication and reported effects and any side-effects;
5. any warning signs that might indicate a relapse of his mental state or repetition of offending behaviour together with the time lapse in which this could occur;
6. a report on present home circumstances; and
7. supervision and after-care arrangements which the hospital considers appropriate and inappropriate in this particular case.

The discharging hospital may also provide details of the circumstances of the offence that led to the patient's admission to hospital and of the legal authority for that admission. In any event, the Home Office will provide this information together with a note of any relevant previous convictions as soon as the name of the social supervisor is known.

It is crucial that the social supervisor has all the above information and hospitals should be challenged when it is not forthcoming. It is not uncommon to encounter cases where only the barest of information has been made available to the distinct disadvantage of the supervisor and ultimately the patient. In cases of difficulty in obtaining relevant information C3 division at the Home Office is always prepared to assist.

Meanwhile, close liaison between the after-care team is essential if supervision is to be effective. The key people will be the supervising psychiatrist, social supervisor, hostel staff and any other person who will be regularly involved in the after-care arrangements. It is important for both nominated supervisors to be involved in the predischarge discussions and have an opportunity to meet and plan their supervisory arrangements jointly. Others such as hostel staff will need to be involved at this stage as well as receiving the appropriate information. It is crucial that all the community personnel work as a team with a common plan of action. There is no room at any stage for individual workers to pursue their own agenda.

The discharge planning arrangements should use the concepts of the care programme approach (D of H, 1990) involving carers and patient. The only real difference is that the patient has no choice but to agree with the after-care arrangements, as they are statutory. Nevertheless, involving the patient at this stage is likely to ensure better compliance and acceptance of the probable intrusiveness of the supervisor when the former is eventually in the community.

The supervisory process

The starting point for the supervisory process with the restricted patient must be to consider its prime purpose. As long ago as 1973 the Aarvold committee (HO/DHSS, 1973) said:

> for a patient whose case has been identified as requiring special care in assessment we consider that the arrangements for supervision and continuing care, which in other cases might entail some compromise between the interests of the patient and of the public should be biased towards satisfaction of the requirements of public safety.

In the subsequent guidance notes for social supervisors (HO/DHSS, 1987a) this philosophy is applied to the supervision of all restricted patients and is summed up in the simple statement: 'The purpose of formal supervision resulting from conditional discharge is to protect the public from further serious harm.'

The guidance notes go on to say that this can be best achieved by:

1. assisting the patient's successful integration into the community after what may have been a long period of detention in hospital under conditions of security; and
2. by close monitoring of the patient's progress so that in the event of subsequent deterioration in the patient's mental health or of a perceived increase in the risk of danger to the public, steps can be taken to assist the patient and protect the public.

A conditional discharge also facilitates the assessment of the patient in the community to enable a decision to be taken as to whether controls may eventually be lifted by way of an absolute discharge.

Clearly, much reliance and responsibility is placed on the shoulders of the social supervisor and it is important that the supervisory task is entered into with a clear sense of purpose and direction. Unlike the supervision of offenders discharged from prison there are no national standards for the supervision of conditionally discharged patients in the community. Recently developed national standards for the former sets out clear requirements to be met in all cases where prisoners are released from custody except in the case of life-sentence prisoners (Home Office, Probation Service Division, 1992). By contrast the guidance notes for social supervisors are just that, apart from certain reporting requirements. It is suggested that although some elements in the role of social supervisor are important if supervision is to be effective in achieving its purpose, the specific requirements of supervision will vary from case to case and over time.

Accordingly, the supervisor will need to have an individual strategy for each supervisee but with some core features which will be applicable to all. Although the patient will have met with the supervisor before discharge and will have been informed of the conditions of his discharge before leaving hospital, it will be helpful to reiterate these details as soon as possible when he is in the community. Face-to-face contact should therefore take place between supervisor and patient, preferably on the day of discharge or as soon as possible thereafter. The supervisor will wish to go over the essential points of the subsequent supervision programme and will probably cover the following:

- the specific requirements of the conditional discharge, e.g. residence at a specified address, regular contact with the social supervisor and supervising psychiatrist;
- limitations on travel away from home area;
- discussion of any anticipated problems;
- information about the social supervisor, supervising psychiatrist, their office addresses and telephone numbers and any other contact points; and
- planned frequency of contact and next appointment.

If as stated in the guidance to social supervisors, 'The protection of the public from serious harm is best assured, in the long run, by their successful integration into the community of the patient,' the focus of the supervisory services particularly in the early stages will need to concentrate on the following:

- need for further rehabilitation;
- retraining opportunities;
- employment prospects;
- daytime activity;
- financial matters;
- social outlets/support;
- family contact; and
- areas of concern.

Supervisors should therefore not only be monitoring the patient's progress but actively promoting a constructive approach to his resettlement in the community. The actual amount of contact required will obviously vary from patient to patient. Although the frequency of meeting is not stipulated in the guidelines, they recommend that there should be a minimum contact of once a week for the first month after discharge, reducing to once a fortnight and then once a month as the social supervisor judges appropriate. Some patients will need considerably more, particularly in the early stages of their discharge.

As the patient makes progress he may wish to make changes to his circumstances such as moving home, taking on a job or even simply having a holiday. Nevertheless, such changes should not be made unilaterally and should always be discussed and agreed by the supervisor first. The prime consideration of the supervisor should always be the risk entailed in making such changes. Normally an absence from home of more than a few days is actively discouraged during the first six months of discharge. An absence of more than two weeks would require the supervisor to notify the appropriate social services department or probation service in the holiday area. A holiday abroad would need Home Office consent.

Where the patient wishes to change his home address, this should be negotiated with the supervisor who will need to write to C3 division, Home Office, to seek agreement to the proposed change. The home address is stipulated on the discharge warrant and will need to be amended accordingly. Similarly, if the supervisor is away from his post for even a short period of time, a collegue should be nominated as a temporary stand-in and the patient and other professionals notified accordingly. Where such an absence extends to two months or more, the Home Office will need to be informed.

The dilemmas of supervision

Although the prime purpose of supervision is to protect the public from serious harm, it is also expected that supervisors have a positive and constructive approach towards the patient's social rehabilitation rather than simply monitoring progress. So although account needs to be taken of public unease, there is often a difficult balance to be drawn between the protection of the public and the rights, welfare and resettlement needs of the patient. On the one hand, the supervisor must act like a 'social policeman' and on the other he must develop a supportive and positive relationship to facilitate the patient's integration into the community. Who then should be the focus of attention; the patient or the community? What implications are there for practice? What style of work needs to be adopted?

In considering the above it must be remembered that this is not an 'ordinary' type of supervision. There are almost as many expectations and limitations of freedom on the supervisor as there are on the patient. In the past the patient has demonstrated by his offence that in certain circumstances he is dangerous, and these circumstances cannot be allowed to recur in the future. This may mean the avoidance of certain types of situations and/or developing the patient's ability to confront them without risk in the future.

The supervisor therefore must be constantly alert to 'situational threats' to the patient or any sign of his deterioration in mental health or social abilities. This means keeping close to the patient, having enough knowledge of the individual and his current situation to identify increasing risks, 'trigger' factors or warning signs. Supervision in this context cannot be a passive activity.

While general social work skills are applicable to the restricted patient, the less directive approach of the more traditional interventions are not always suitable. There may also be a need to take a more controlling and assertive stance (Floud and Young, 1981). In other words, supervisors must adopt what Prins describes as an 'intrusive' style of supervision (Prins, 1990a). He highlights the need to develop a high threshold of suspiciousness with a concern for great attention to detail. This means developing a capacity for asking the 'unimaginable', 'unaskable' and 'unthinkable' questions. Above all, supervisors must be sensitive to 'history repeating itself' in terms of the patient's risk profile. This is often more clearly identified in retrospect, sometimes with tragic results when missed, as illustrated by the following example:

Case study

Henry, aged 29, was admitted to a special hospital with a diagnosis of personality disorder and depressive illness. His admission offence was the stabbing to death of his authoritarian mother during an argument. After six years he was conditionally discharged into the community to a supervised hostel and attended a local day hospital on a daily basis. Tragically, after three months attendance he stabbed the nursing sister in charge of the day hospital following an altercation. In reviewing the incident following recall to hospital, the clinical team discovered that the victim had been a woman of the same age, stature and disposition as Henry's mother. At the time of the second stabbing Henry had again become depressed and argumentative. The day hospital sister had become a surrogate victim.

This case illustrates the vital importance of receiving adequate information about the patient's background and offence on discharge, understanding the nature and circumstances of the index offence, and being alert to the deterioration in the patient's mental health and the development of a potentially dangerous situation. Moreover, the supervisor needs to know what to look for. In the case quoted above, any female with authority over the patient may have been at risk and the victim could just as easily have been the hostel warden who was also a middle-aged woman. Had this type of risk being identified earlier, guidance could have been given on the handling of the patient's argumentative behaviour in order to avoid confrontations.

In order to properly monitor the patient's demeanour and lifestyle it is necessary to have regular access to his living accommodation, including his bedroom. The pictures, posters, contents, arrangement, etc. will carry many indications of the more private aspects of his life and thought processes. Prins (1990b) makes the point that had those responsible for Graham Young's supervision (the case quoted at the beginning of this chapter on page 140) gained access to his living accommodation they would have found rich pictorial evidence of an ongoing sinister preoccupation with poisons and death. Such 'intrusiveness' may be one of the few opportunities of gaining access to the patient's fantasy life. This 'inner world' is difficult to penetrate, yet it provides valuable insights into the stability of the patient and the possible future risk to the public.

A further danger to be wary of is to indulge in what Prins describes as 'rescue operations; that is to believe uncritically that the only thing the client or patient requires is to be 'rescued' from the iniquitous system' (Prins, 1990a). Such action results in the worker engaging in the process of 'denial' to the extent that negative reports from the patient and others are not 'heard' and eventually not given. To accept such information about lack of progress or worse would indicate a failure on the part of the 'rescuer' and so it is better not to receive it.

Statements made by the patient, therefore, may need to be double-checked, presumptions challenged and current behaviour patterns compared with previous ones. Failure to be appraised with all the facts, to monitor with persistence, to ask probing questions, in short to intrude into the patient's life, is likely to result in loose supervision which is open to exploitation.

One such tragic case is that of a Daniel Mudd who, having been admitted to Broadmoor at sixteen-and-a-half for a non-homicide case, was subsequently conditionally discharged five years later. For three years his life in the community became increasingly chaotic and finally resulted in him killing a woman living in a hostel. The enquiry that followed concluded that Mr Mudd's accounts of his behaviour were accepted without challenge, no links were made between past and present offending patterns and that the five sets of files held by the local authority were never collated or screened effectively (Wiltshire County Council, 1988).

It is clear that the supervisor should certainly know of, if not be involved in, all areas of the patient's life. This should involve disappointments as well as achievements. One area of difficulty is likely to be in connection with employment. For a person with either a psychiatric or criminal background, finding work is a problem. Few employers are sympathetic to either group and the offender/patient is doubly disadvantaged. While offender/patients should not be dishonest in the information they give to potential employers, the amount of detail given may determine whether the job is secured or not. The question is often whether to disclose or not disclose the fact that the patient is a conditionally discharged restricted patient and whether details of the offence are relevant. Obviously, a patient with a history of offences against children should not be seeking employment in a childcare setting, but in many cases there will be room for discretion.

Although the patient himself may decide on the level of disclosure or even whether to disclose at all, the responsibility to decide what information to disclose and to whom is the social supervisor's. The only exception is where medical information is concerned where the supervising psychiatrist has the responsibility. It is suggested, however, in the supervisors' guidelines that any disclosure of information to a third party should be done with the agreement of the patient. Disclosures against the patient's wishes should only be done if there are strong, overriding reasons for doing so. Interestingly, research into the integration of special hospital patients into the community showed a significant association between levels of disclosure and the number of incidents and successful integration (Norris, 1984). Secretive behaviour or 100% disclosures were less likely to be 'incident' free with those patients making disclosures with some discretion being less frequently involved in 'incidents' (such as psychiatric symptoms, assaults, further offences, return to hospital). Norris concluded that 'The insistence of some supervisors that patients should always disclose their backgrounds seems excessive and it is likely to undermine self-esteem. As time goes by it may be more important to think of reducing all sources of stigma for the patient.' It is suggested, therefore, that the necessity to always disclose, especially over time, may be humiliating. A patient's decision to disclose but not indiscriminately may be a sign of increasing self-confidence and successful integration.

Teamwork

Many of the issues discussed above will apply equally to others involved in caring for and supervising the patient in the community, particularly hostel staff and the supervising psychiatrist. Nevertheless, it is the social supervisor who is the key worker with responsibility for ensuring that effective liaison takes place. This should also involve the general practitioner, community psychiatric nurse and daycare staff as appropriate. Although all are important, perhaps the most crucial link will be between the social supervisor and the supervising psychiatrist. As stated in the guidelines for supervising psychiatrists, 'the two most important elements in effective supervision are the development of a close relationship with the patient and the maintenance of a good liaison with the social supervisor' (HO/DHSS, 1987b).

Teamwork and communication are key factors highlighted by Prins in any work with offender/patients (Prins, 1983). He stresses the importance of mutual support, sharing of tasks and giving up notions of 'going it alone'. Thus such liaison will begin at the predischarge stage and both parties will agree a common overall approach to the patient's treatment and reintegration into the community with a clear understanding of how they will communicate effectively after discharge. Both the supervising psychiatrist and the social supervisor are also required to report to the Home Office on the patient's condition one month after discharge and every three months thereafter. Copies of such reports should be sent to each, with an expectation of regularly discussing the patient's situation and reviewing progress. In doing so, the social supervisor will have the benefit of additional knowledge of progress gained from employers, friends, family and any other relevant people.

Change of social supervisor

In cases where serious offences have been committed the Home Secretary requires active supervision and reporting to be kept up for at least five years. In less serious cases it has to have been maintained for at least two years. Inevitably, therefore, there will be changes in social supervisor, perhaps on several occasions. Research carried out in the early 1980s showed that the average length of supervision by the same supervisor was less than two years with 20% lasting less than six months (Norris, 1984). Such changes are uncomfortable if not detrimental to the patient. Continuity of supervision permits the establishment of a relationship which has been found to contribute to positive integration into the community. There appears to be an association between good support between supervisor and patient and successful resettlement. A change of supervisor is therefore potentially disruptive and Norris' research showed that patients found such changes unsettling. In particular, they disliked having to recall their past history every time their supervisor changed.

The supervisors' guidelines recognized that a change of supervisor may be upsetting for the patient and stresses that care should be taken to ease the transition. It also recommends that the outgoing supervisor passes his successor full information about the case and supplements this with an oral briefing. Furthermore, full discussion and handover should be effected with the others involved in the patient's care. Unfortunately, this does not always happen. Both research and experience has shown that difficulties of transfer of information are commonplace and that the quality and consistency of supervision is diluted at each change. It is imperative therefore that such disruption is minimized to prevent important information about the patient's needs being lost. In the case of Daniel Mudd, quoted earlier in the chapter, the social supervisor left at the crucial time of Mr Mudd moving into his own flat where he would receive no immediate day-to-day supervision. Not only was there no preparation for transfer, but a gap of one month elapsed before another supervisor was appointed (Wiltshire County Council, 1988).

Recall

Despite all the efforts of those involved, there will be occasions, currently about 55 per year, when a recall to hospital is necessary. If there is any concern at all about the patient's mental state or behaviour, all the professionals involved will need to discuss the situation and consider the best way forward. In particular, where the social supervisor has concerns for the safety of the patient or others he should contact the supervising psychiatrist immediately. In addition a report to the Home Office should always be made in a case in which:

1. there appears to be an actual or potential risk to the public;
2. contact with the patient is lost or the patient is unwilling to co-operate with supervision;
3. the patient's behaviour or condition suggest a need for further in-patient treatment in hospital; and
4. the patient is charged with or convicted of an offence.

However, even in the event of the above, recall to the discharging hospital may not always be the most productive way of dealing with the situation. In some cases, a brief admission to the local psychiatric hospital may be all that is required to stabilize a patient whose mental health has deteriorated. The supervising psychiatrist has the authority to make a local decision to arrange such an admission, preferably on an informal basis. If it is not possible to secure the patient's co-operation in this process, then it may be necessary to consider using civil powers such as those under Sections 2, 3 or 4 of the Mental Health Act 1983. In other cases where the anti-social behaviour may be unconnected with mental disorder, the patient can be dealt with as necessary by the normal processes under the criminal law. If a non-custodial sentence is imposed the terms of the previous conditional discharge will continue and the supervisors should resume their role. Where the court imposes a sentence of imprisonment, the Home Secretary will usually refrain from deciding what further action to take until the patient nears the end of his prison sentence.

The Home Secretary's decision to issue a recall order will depend on the patient's previous history and current risk to the public. Where the patient has shown himself capable of serious violence in the past, fairly minor irregularities in behaviour or failure to co-operate in the supervisory process may be enough reason for recall. Conversely, where there is no history of serious risk, such action may be unnecessary unless there are current indications of a probable physical danger to others. If a recall to hospital is authorized, the patient is once again detained as a restricted patient under the legal authority which applied before the conditional discharge.

Where a patient has been recalled to hospital, certain procedures are to be followed to ensure that he understands the reasons for recall and is reminded of his statutory rights under the Mental Health Act 1983. A local authority circular issued in April 1993 clearly sets out the procedures to be followed (Department of Health, 1993):

Stage 1: The person returning the patient to hospital (who may be a probation officer or approved social worker) should inform him in simple terms that he is being recalled to hospital by the Home Secretary under Section 42(3) of the Mental Health Act 1983 and that to the extent that this is possible, a further explanation will be given later. The reason(s) for recalling the patient should be explained to ther nearest relative, if one is available, within 72 hours.

Stage 2: An explanation should be given to the patient of the reason(s) for his recall as soon as possible after re-admission to hospital and in any event within 72 hours. This should be done by the responsible medical officer or deputy, an approved social worker, or an appropriate administrator representing the hospital managers. The person giving the explanation should ensure, so far as the patient's mental condition allows, that the patient understands the reason(s).

Stage 3: a written explanation of the reasons for recall should be provided for that patient within 72 hours of being readmitted to the hospital. Written information on the reason(s) should also be given to the patient's nearest relative (subject to the patient's consent).

The social supervisor is probably best placed to liaise with the family and offer whatever support may be necessary. They will also need to be informed of the patient's right to apply to the Mental Health Review Tribunal. In any event, the Home Secretary has the statutory duty under Section 75(a) to refer the case to a Tribunal within one month of recall. At such hearings the Home Secretary, in preparing his statement for the Tribunal, is likely to draw on reports received from supervisors. The supervisors may also be asked to appear at the Tribunal hearing.

Termination of supervision

In a minority of cases a conditionally discharged patient is subject to a restriction order of specified duration. When the nominated date has been reached he is automatically absolutely discharged from all restrictions or liability for recall. In most cases, however, the restriction order is for an indefinite period and its lifting is dependent on the recommendations by the supervising officers and agreement by the Home Secretary. It is not uncommon for the psychiatric supervision to be lifted some time before the social supervision in cases where the safety of the public would not be at risk if the patient ceased to receive psychiatric oversight. Social supervision, on the other hand, is likely to be more protracted and lasts for a minimum of five years where the index offence was serious.

The key factor, as always, is the element of risk to the public if supervision were to be lifted. The guidelines for social supervisors state, 'The Home Secretary will wish to see evidence of a prolonged period of stability in the community which has been tested by a variety of normal pressures and experiences.' In other words, the supervisor will need to feel convinced that, if repeated, the specific pressures and experiences which provoked the index offence will no longer be a cause for concern. In considering the patient's readiness for absolute discharge it is useful to see if and how the prime tasks of social supervision have been fulfilled:

1. assisting in the patient's successful integration into the community;
2. closely monitoring the patient's progress; and
3. assessment of the patient in the community.

A case study will serve to illustrate the exercise:

Case study

Paul, an epileptic since birth, had a difficult childhood and adolescence being described as easily led and immature. As a teenager he began to commit a number of petty offences and eventually received a short prison sentence for burglary. On release from prison he quicky got into trouble, fighting, disturbing the peace, etc., and finally set fire to a warehouse where he had a part-time job, causing thousands of pounds worth of damage. This occurred after being sacked for insubordination and breaking up with his girlfriend. He was subsequently admitted to a special hospital with a diagnosis of personality disorder and mental impairment. After six years he was transferred to a local psychiatric hospital and a year later, at the age of 29, he was conditionally discharged into the community.

Initially after discharge there was much work for the social supervisor in helping Paul to integrate into the community. For the first year he was seen on a weekly basis and closely supervised in a staffed hostel. He was enabled to attend a work-therapy unit five days a week where he also received life-skills and social-skills training. Gradually he established some friendships and had a few girlfriends. After about 18 months he moved into his own accommodation and was able to look after himself. However, the first two years after discharge were not without difficulties. There were the occasional crises at work when he lost his temper following minor altercations and he sometimes walked out. Only the intervention and support of the social supervisor stopped him being barred from the sheltered work placement. When he started living on his own, he also initially became isolated and lonely. Again the social supervisor intervened to seek suitable social outlets and arrange a reintroduction to family contact. On one occasion Paul became engaged but when the relationship broke up he became clinically depressed, requiring intervention from the supervising psychiatrist.

Nevertheless, after a lot of hard work by Paul and his social supervisor, he gradually managed to control his temper and his work improved. He spent more time in outside employment and eventually got a full-time job with a local builders' merchant. His relationship with his family slowly became re-established and he acquired another steady girlfriend.

The social supervisor worked very hard in helping to establish Paul in the community, especially in the first two years. The marks of integration were independent accommodation, steady employment, social outlets and stable relationships. Because the supervisor closely monitored the situation initially with weekly contact and more often when necessary, early signs of difficulty were nipped in the bud and hurdles overcome. After five years the social supervisor felt confident enough about Paul's stabilty to recommend an absolute discharge to the Home Office. By examining detailed notes of how Paul had reacted to difficulties in the past and comparing them with a much more positive record in the last two-and-a-half years, it was possible to demonstrate that progress had been made. For example, despite further disagreements at work, Paul had not lost his temper or walked out. Although a relationship of twelve months standing with a girlfriend came to an end, he was upset but did not become clinically depressed. His self-care skills had developed significantly and he had the confidence to seek his own social outlets. In short, there was enough evidence to support the application for absolute discharge which was finally accepted. It should be added that an absolute discharge does not preclude continuing contact between the patients and the supervisors on a non-statutory basis.

The other avenue for applying for an absolute discharge is through the Mental Health Review Tribunal. The Tribunal has power either to direct a variation of the conditions attached to discharge or to direct an absolute discharge.

Support for the social supervisor

Few social workers or probation officers have much experience of supervising patients subject to special restrictions in the community. Probation officers are perhaps better prepared for the task by virtue of their experience in dealing with offenders released from custody on licence, although the added dimensins of mental illness and potential dangerousness cannot be minimized.

With only 600–700 restricted patients being supervised in the community at any one time, the expertise and knowledge in working with this group is thinly spread. Accordingly, the stress and feelings of isolation experienced by social supervisors should be recognized by the agencies concerned. Even with close supervision and support there will be periods of high anxiety and feelings of vulnerability. The very nature of some of the offences committed by patients are outside the realms of 'normal' experience. The perceived potential for disaster if the supervisor 'gets it wrong' can be a frightening situation to be in. Indeed, as Prins says, 'there is certainly little doubt that the way in which some offenders present themselves to us can fill us with an intangible disquiet and even apprehension' (Prins, 1986). It is a task that can be onerous and emotionally demanding and one that needs a capacity to examine one's own motives and understanding.

This is a task that cannot be undertaken alone. Although there may be support and collaboration with the other professionals involved in the patient's care, it is no replacement for good, sound supervision. The supervisor must seek out the worker's blind spots, must challenge denial and must ensure that the uncomfortable, 'unaskable' questions are pursued. There can be no room for complacency even if the alternative is unpalatable. Such support should be provided by more experienced colleagues although they themselves are not immune from the anxieties of dealing with uncertain, ambiguous situations. Line managers will have their own fears and fantasies, and as well as the intervention of the immediate supervisor to the patient, progress in a case is often clearly determined by those giving support and supervisory back-up (HM Inspectorate of Probation and Home Office, 1987).

SUMMARY

Social workers have a key role to play in secure psychiatric institutions in terms of assessment throughcare, rehabilitation and resettlement. Most important is the need to maintain the patient's links with the outside world, particularly with his family. Families themselves will also need much help in coming to terms with the events that led to the patient's original detention.

On discharge the patient will have enormous needs for support and supervision and the social supervisor needs adequate preparation for the task. The social supervision of restricted patients requires an assertive, intrusive style of work coupled with a sensitive approach to the use of authority. Good teamwork and liaison with other professionals and across agencies is crucial, as is the need for first-class supervision and support.

REFERENCES

Baxter, R. (1991) The mentally disordered offender in hospital: the role of the Home Office, in *The Mentally Disordered Offender* (eds K. Herbst and J. Gunn), Butterworth-Heinemann, Oxford, pp. 132–44.

Dell, S. (1980) *The Transfer of Special Hospital Patients to National Health Service Hospitals*, Special Hospitals Research Report No. 16, Special Hospitals Research Unit, London.

Department of Health (1990) *The Care Programme Approach (CPA) for People with a Mental Illness Referred to the Specialist Psychiatric Services* HC(90)/LASSL (90) 11, Department of Health, London.

Department of Health (1993) *Recall of Mentally Disordered Patients Subject to Home Office Restrictions on Discharge* Local Authority Circular LAC (1993) 9, Department of Health, London.

Floud, J. and Young, W.(1981) *Dangerousness and Criminal Justice*, Heinemann Educational Books, London.

Hamilton, J. (1990) Special hospitals and the state hospital, in *Principles and Practice of Forensic Psychiatry* (eds R. Bluglass and P. Bowden), Churchill Livingstone, Edinburgh, pp. 1363–73.

HM Inspectorate of Probation and Home Office (1987) *Issues for Senior Management in the Supervision of Dangerous and High Risk Offenders* HMSO, London.

Home Office and Department of Health and Social Security (1973) *Report of the Review of Procedures for the Discharge and Supervision of Psychiatric Patients Subject to Special Restrictions*, (The Aarvold Report), Cmnd 5191, HMSO, London.

Home Office and Department of Health and Social Security (1987a) *Mental Health Act 1983 Supervision and After Care of Conditionally Discharged Restricted Patients: Notes for the Guidance of Social Supervisors*, Home Office, London.

Home Office and Department of Health and Social Security (1987b) *Mental Health Act 1983 Supervision and After-Care of Conditionally Discharged Restricted Patients: Notes for the Guidance of Supervising Psychiatrists*, Home Office, London.

Home Ofice and Department of Health and Social Security (1987c) *Mental Health Act 1983 Supervision and After Care of Conditionally Discharged Restricted Patients: Notes for the Guidance of Hospitals Preparing for the Conditional Discharge of Restricted Patients*, Home Office, London.

Home Office Probation Service Division (1992) *National Standards for the Supervision of Offenders in the Community*, HMSO, London.

Mace, A.E. (1991) A probation service perspective, in *The Mentally Disordered Offender* (eds K. Herbst and J. Gunn), Butterworth-Heinemann, Oxford, pp. 196–205.

Marchant, C. (1993) Secure hospitals. *Community Care*, 2 September 14–15.

Mental Health Act Commission (1987) *Biennial Report 1985–1987*, HMSO, London.

Norris, M. (1984) *Integration of special Hospital Patients into the Community* Gower Publishing, Aldershot.

Prins, H. (1983) The care of the psychiatric prisoner – discharge into the community and its implications. *Medicine, Science and the Law*, Vol. 23, No. 2, 79–86.

Prins, H. (1986) *Dangerous Behaviour: the Law and Mental Disorder*, Tavistock, London.

Prins, H. (1990a) The supervision of potentially dangerous offender patients in England and Wales. *International Journal of Offender Therapy and Comparative Criminology*, **34**, Dec (3), 213–21.

Prins, H. (1990b) Some observations on the supervision of dangerous offender patients. *British Journal of Psychiatry*, **156**, 157–62.

Steadman, H.J. and Cocozza, J.J. (1974) *Careers of the Criminally Insane*, Lexington Books, Lexington.

Vaughan, P.J. (1979) The key to the growth of social work in Broadmoor. *Health and Social Service Journal*, 6 April, 384–6.

Vaughan, P.J. (1980) Letters and visits to long-stay Broadmoor patients. *British Journal of Social Work*, **10**, 471–81.

Vaughan, P.J. and Fortt, C. (1983) The differing role of the social worker in the special hospital/penal setting. *Prison Service Journal*, April, 17–19.

Wiltshire County Council (1988) *Report Of A Departmental Enquiry Into The Discharge Of Responsibilities By The Wiltshire Social Services In Relation To Daniel Mudd From His Release From Broadmoor In May 1983 Until His Arrest In December 1986 For The Murder Of Ruth Perrett*, Trowbridge, Wilts.

7

Residential and daycare services

If community care is to be a real and positive alternative to in-patient care, it must include a range of residential and daycare services. The depth and span of this range is partly a function of levels of funding at national and local level, but since this is not likely to be under the influence of either the readers or writers of this book this constraint will not be further discussed. Other crucial determinants of what is offered by way of community care are the vision, energy and commitment of staff who plan and deliver residential and daycare services for offenders and the mentally disordered. These staff may be working for social service departments, the probation service, the health service or in the voluntary and private sectors. Paid, trained staff are likely to be the key personnel in making major decisions about referrals and the ethos of the unit or centre, but this is also an area of work where untrained staff and volunteers can and do make a crucial contribution.

Community care for the mentally disordered offender presents a particular challenge because the numbers involved are relatively small. As a result there is rarely a case to be made for a hostel or daycentre which deals exclusively with this client group. The exception to this might be provision for a specialist bail hostel in a large city such as London. Smith (1993) makes just this case because of the reluctance of most bail hostels to accept referrals of mentally disordered offenders. In the main, however, fieldworkers are faced with making referrals to hostels and daycentres where staff may lack the experience of working with the client group and so be fearful and reluctant to accept this type of referral. Persuasion, education and persistence may all be required to obtain a service that another client might receive without difficulty.

A second range of difficulties arise from mentally disordered offenders having membership of two client groups for whom community services are potentially funded by three different organizations: namely, social services departments, the probation service and the National Health Service. Recent changes in the health service mean that this is becoming fragmented into a range of trusts, and social services are currently threatened with changes to unitary authorities likely to be considerably smaller than existing local authorities. Some probation services will probably amalgamate to cover larger authorities, possibly with boundaries aligned with police authorities. The net result for a small, doubly stigmatized group such as mentally disordered offenders is likely to be official neglect. The obvious danger is that financial advantage for any one organization will combine with individual prejudice and reluctance to offer services to this group with the rationale that the client is properly the responsibility of another organization. What is needed on the fieldwork side to improve this situation are case managers with the knowledge and experience of working with this client group, working from an organizational base that straddles at least the boundaries between social services and the probation service. Such is the case in Scotland but even there the boundary with the health service remains a source of difficulty.

On the residential and daycare side there may be a need for specialist hostels and centres but the reality is that this will remain the exception rather than the rule. This means that the challenge is for mainstream mental health and probation hostels and daycentres to include provision for this client group within their brief. It seems that there are difficulties in making this a reality and this chapter seeks to address some of those obstacles. Residential and daycare services are commonly treated together but in reality they provide rather different challenges as places of work and so will be discussed separately. However, the same major topics will be discussed for both settings so the material will be presented in parallel, under the common headings of Tasks and functions, Referrals, Ethos and Discharge.

TASKS AND FUNCTIONS

Residential services

Hostels are often staffed by untrained workers on low wages working with staff-to-resident ratios that are poor compared to the childcare field. These staff are expected to cope with a wide variety of people including some who may be difficult to manage because of their personalities, mental disorder or offending behaviour. The mismatch between the difficulty of the task and the rewards and support available to those undertaking it reveals the depth of muddled thinking and unreasonable expectations that has surrounded residential work for many years. It is a confusion that is unlikely to go away as there is little evidence that the demanding nature of residential work is going to be widely recognized and the lot of the worker improved in terms of status, salary and training. However, it is important to state at the outset that this is a difficult job that should be better paid and highly valued and that it would be far more manageable if staffing levels were improved and specialist training made available.

This is not necessarily true of all forms of residential work, particularly where a hostel is essentially providing long-term accommodation for those who cannot manage fully independent living in the community. It is, however, true for those hostels that provide an immediate alternative to prison or psychiatric in-patient care. In such establishments it is common to find staff coping with people who may have recently committed serious crimes, whose mental state is agitated and who may be emotionally labile. To care for people through such periods of crisis and distress requires a blend of therapeutic and controlling interventions. If this is to be effective, adequate levels of staffing and clarity of purpose are essential.

Having established that residential work is an unrecognized but demanding job, what more can be said about its purposes which will improve community care of the mentally disordered offender? The first point to be made is that those responsible for a hostel need to be clear about its purposes and to make a link between those purposes and crucial issues such as staffing levels, types of staff required, training and consultancy.

If, for example, a probation hostel is receiving referrals of mentally disordered offenders the management group needs to consider carefully how to respond to this. If it is agreed that such referrals will be accepted, then there is work to be done to help staff to feel ready to respond to this challenge. This may include some work on fears and prejudices about mental disorder (see Chapter Three for some ideas about this) but it should also involve developing closer relationships with mental health services locally so that advice on such matters as management, administration of drugs and psychiatric symptomatology can be available to staff when they need it. Thought should also be given to whether psychiatric nursing qualifications should be included as desirable or essential requirements when the next staff vacancy occurs. Better still, additional staff could be recruited with this professional experience and expertise. This will increase costs, so arguments will need to be mounted about the fees to be charged or the levels of funding that need to be sought.

Similarly, a mental health hostel that is considering the possibility of taking referrals of those with a history of offending may need to think about the sorts of admission 'contracts' they develop so that supervising probation officers as well as potential residents themselves are clear about the consequences of re-offending. A contract may also help secure a better level of visiting and support from the probation officer.

Assuming that the management of the hostel has bitten on the bullet and faced that taking mentally disordered offenders into the unit will require thought and planning, a further set of considerations are likely to emerge about the primary task of the hostel. Miller and Gwynne (1972) carried out a study of units for people with physical disabilities and identified two approaches to the care of the residents which they called the 'horticultural' and 'warehousing' models. The horticultural model, as its name implies, was concerned for the growth and development of residents, while the warehousing model paid attention to ensuring the physical comfort and care of residents. Most residential workers are likely to identify with the horticultural model, with its promise and hope of change, but the authors' analysis demands more thought than this 'gut reaction'. They point out that the horticultural model fits well with the task of maximizing the independence of those who have previously lacked adequate emotional, practical and technical support to achieve this. However, a growth model does not sit comfortably with meeting the needs of someone in the last stages of a degenerative disease. For residents such as this, the main need is for high quality physical and emotional care in order to conserve as much energy as possible for activities and relationships that will probably be more important than physical independence.

The key therefore is to achieve an assessment of the needs of the resident that is unclouded by the wishes and needs of the staff group. This is not at all easy and Miller and Gwynne deliberately use the emotive labels of horticultural and warehousing to confront staff attitudes and particularly staff defences against the anxiety of caring for people who are not getting better. The danger is that some staff will find this reality unbearable and so will impose a horticultural model on those for whom it is inappropriate. If residents' needs can be assessed without undue distortion by staff needs and defences, then it is but a small step to match the way the hostel is organized around the primary task. This is no simple task, however, and it is a recurring challenge for managers to stay in touch with the primary task and to enable the staff group to do the same. To achieve this, it is hard to overestimate the importance of an external consultant to the staff group.

An important strand in Miller and Gwynne's analysis is the link between attitudes and values in wider society towards disabled people and the nature of the primary task that residential workers are expected to fulfil on behalf of that society. It is not difficult to extend this values approach to working with the mentally disordered offender. Social attitudes vary from the totally punitive, 'Lock them up and throw away the key', to the distantly tolerant, 'Not in my back yard' response. In either case, society is sending an essentially negative message and inevitably some of this will rub off on the workers. The only positive aspect that might be discerned in societal attitudes towards the care of this client group is admiration and a degree of fascination for those who are willing to share their lives with people whose behaviour is seen as being outside normal bounds. This is evident in attitudes towards such people as psychiatric nurses in special hospitals. Even this cachet is only available to those working with serious offenders: the less notorious minor offenders provide little social status!

Miller and Gwynne's models of care can be usefully applied to the task of providing for the needs of the mentally disordered offender living in a hostel, though perhaps the term 'maintenance' could be substituted in place of warehousing. For those with a history of psychotic illness the primary need may be for high-quality maintenance in which there is regular activity and attention to medication, active monitoring of levels of functioning and a concern to avoid high levels of expressed emotion. For others, where personality disorder is a predominant issue, a horticultural model could well be appropriate with an emphasis on personality development and changing attitudes. However, more thought needs to be given to the question of what anxieties staff may be defending themselves against, as these are most likely to get in the way of the fulfilment of the primary task.

Pursuing the logic that underlies this book, there are probably some common anxieties related to this group and these relate to dangerousness and unpredictability. Responses to these anxieties vary along a continuum from total control to denial of the seriousness of the risk posed by the individual. Special hospitals with their emphasis on security and surveillance represent one extreme, while denial is exemplified by the community care of some patently dangerous individuals who are placed in unsupervised situations. The case of Christopher Clunis appears to be an example of the latter (Ritchie *et al.*, 1994). A balanced approach is needed, based on a realistic assessment of the dangers posed. Fundamental is sufficient staff on duty so that responsibility can be shared and the needs of all residents met. If this is not available there is a realistic worry that preoccupation with the mentally disordered offender resident will distract staff and skew the work of the hostel.

In addition to this general concern with safety and dangerousness, there are also likely to be particular anxieties for some groups, for example, probation hostel staff may well have major concerns arising from lack of experience of mental disorder. This may manifest itself in treating mentally disordered offenders as if they were the same as all other offenders and so making no allowance for their mental state.

On the other hand, they may overreact to the label of mentally disordered offender and treat all such referrals as equally dangerous or unpredictable. What is needed is an approach that finds the middle ground between these two positions and allows informed decision-making and management to take place.

Assuming that such a middle position has been achieved, there still remains a major difficulty for staff. This is that it is not uncommon to find residents with different needs in the same establishment and the challenge then is to devise an approach that allows these varied sets of needs to be met. However, hostels with a strong commitment to personal growth and development, using group psychotherapy, psychodrama and the like, may well have to ensure that potential residents who need good quality 'maintenance' are not admitted. The pressures to fill vacancies, particularly for those in the voluntary and private sectors, may make this more difficult in practice than it appears on paper!

The final consideration under this section on Tasks and Functions is that of control and monitoring. Management and staff need to be clear that a control and monitoring function is inescapable with mentally disordered offenders and to consider how this can best be achieved. One danger is that a strict probation hostel approach will be adopted, such as using breach proceedings for those who do not comply with hostel rules. Though the need to hold residents responsible for their behaviour does not disappear with mentally disordered offenders, it does need to be informed by an understanding of the interlock between mental disorder and offending. Where such a link is apparent, it will be more useful and humane to look for psychiatric intervention rather than breach proceedings in order to re-establish the boundaries of acceptable behaviour in the hostel.

The other obvious danger, which is more likely to occur in a mental health hostel, is that insufficient attention will be given to offending behaviour and too much allowance made for individual rule-breaking. Untrained and inexperienced staff need support to face the reality that action must be taken if rules are ignored and the law broken. Experience of using the powers of the court is rare for the staff of mental health hostels compared with those in probation settings, though the sanction of asking the resident to leave does remain. The conflict for staff of rejecting those they seek to help is a recurrent one in these situations. With the resident who presents a real danger to self or others but is not 'sectionable' there is the added dilemma that making the hostel a safer or more orderly place can be achieved by requiring the resident to leave. However, if this cannot be done in a planned way the risk is that this will put members of the general public at risk. Such a scenario should not occur with someone who is under local supervision but there are many individuals not covered by such provision who still raise major concerns if they are not being monitored in the community.

Daycare

Daycentres are an important part of community care for all groups, offering as they do a place to go, something to do, food and companionship for many isolated individuals who are unlikely to find such essentials of human existence elsewhere. By providing such services, they not only meet some of the needs of vulnerable people but also support carers such as families and friends. All these general functions hold good for mentally disordered offenders.

However, some important additional considerations apply in relation to mentally disordered offenders and these relate to the importance of monitoring and the need to accept a degree of social control as an inevitable concommitant of accepting some responsibility for a mentally disordered offender. One way of thinking about the challenge this poses is to view any one attendance at a daycentre as involving an admission and a discharge phase. How the person arrives, whether they are late or early, dishevelled or neat, talkative or silent: all these provide important information about how the person is faring in the community. Anyone working in such a centre needs to pick up such clues and make sure that they or someone else better placed explores the person's situation to see if there is a need for some action. The whole process of the day or session should be informed by the awareness that a discharge will take place within hours. For example, enquiries may need to be made to ascertain if someone has lost his lodgings and is sleeping rough. This can take time, so a decision to start such enquiries needs to be taken sooner rather than later.

To assert this is easy but it is unlikely to happen unless the centre is organized to fulfil this function. If staff and volunteers do not have enough information about those attending to know who they should be actively monitoring it is difficult for them to make a contribution to the task. Reluctance to share confidential information with volunteers is not uncommon and for good reason. A balance has to be found between a person's right to privacy and the worker's (whether paid or voluntary) need to know. Effective monitoring requires teamwork and that is difficult without trust and the sharing of some information.

Teamwork and sharing information may happen spontaneously and this will probably be sufficient in relation to hearing about major events, but it would be unwise to rely on this for regular monitoring and sharing of information. If this is to be done well then regular reviews of the progress of all those attending the centre are important. Care managers may require this as part of monitoring a care package and many establishments will have some sort of system in place. Periodic formal reviews should build on a habit of informal sharing and reviewing at the end of each session. This may be a brief meeting over a cup of tea but it is important that it takes place and that as many workers as possible gather together. Such gatherings often allow crucial bits of the jigsaw to be put together. This is particularly important where a large number of activities are available and it is difficult for any one person to know everything that is going on. It is also important that some senior staff attend this meeting as they have the responsibility for recognizing the significance of the information being shared, for acting on it if necessary and for recording it in some way.

REFERRALS

Residential care

Hostels vary greatly in their referral procedures. Probation hostels commonly accept referrals over the telephone with further information to follow later (often after the person has arrived) while some mental health hostels have elaborate referral forms and procedures involving preliminary visits and trial periods. With such variations reflecting such different patterns of service demand, it is difficult to make useful generalizations but some observations may be helpful.

Even if referrals are accepted over the telephone, it is possible and indeed essential to institute a systematic gathering of information. This is most easily set out in some sort of pro-forma and this is common practice. However, it is also common practice for mentally disordered offenders to be turned down at this stage so the process repays some review. Such referrals are probably being turned down in principle rather than on the merits of the case, so procedures need to be such that sufficient information is gathered to enable a full picture to be obtained. Probation hostel staff may need to review their pro-formas to see if they facilitate the gaining of mental health history, such as current psychiatric diagnosis, current treatment, the number of hospital admissions, the date of last admission.

For mental health hostels, where referral procedures tend to be lengthier, the collection of information may be somewhat easier but the decision-making more complicated. Assessing the likelihood and dangers of re-offending are not necessarily skills to be found in mental health hostels and there may be understandable reluctance to become involved in this demanding area of work. If the management has clarified that this is an area of work that will be covered, the necessary staffing, training and support services should be in place. Fundamental to this work is the advice of an experienced probation officer and ideally such a person should be involved with admission decisions.

A very real danger is that pressure from referral agents and/or the existence of vacancies will lead to the acceptance of a referral against the better judgement of all concerned. With the more serious mentally disordered offenders, i.e. those under social supervision, it is necessary to take account of the guidelines from the Home Office and Department of Health and Social Security (1987) and these are worth thinking about for all referrals of this kind. They include the following concerns:

Should the person come to this area?

It is important to consider this question in deciding whether a person should return to their home town or area, or whether this should be avoided. The latter might be the case if his offences related to family or friends and/or where local attitudes to his offences might make rehabilitation difficult if not impossible. Consideration also needs to be given to the person's own preferences and to the level of support available in terms of employment, daycare, psychiatric and leisure services.

Should the person come to this hostel?

The location of the hostel will obviously be a consideration in relation to the concerns outlined above. Location may also be significant in terms of the specific offences committed by the individual: for example, someone with a history of offences against women would probably not be well-placed in a hostel near accommodation for female nurses. Similar consideration needs to be given to the staffing of the hostel to see if it fits with the perceived needs of the mentally disordered offender. The size of the hostel and the current mix of residents also need to be included in the equation. Prosaic and common-sensical as these criteria may seem, there is good reason to believe they are not always followed. The enquiry into Daniel Mudd's discharge and supervision arrangements (Wiltshire County Council, 1988) revealed little resistance from hostel staff to the proposed admission of a young man who had been in Broadmoor for five years. This was despite the reality that the hostel was mixed, unsupervised by night and predominantly staffed by women. The enquiry records that Daniel Mudd made one resident pregnant and accepted no responsibility for the woman or her child, received warnings for entering the rooms of female residents without invitation and was often the worse for drink. Despite this he was recommended for discharge to his own accommodation and having squandered all his furniture and equipment grant he returned to the hostel for a Christmas party and later that night killed one of the female residents.

Ethnic monitoring

A final point about admission procedures is the importance of gathering information about race and ethnicity. The data reviewed in Chapter Three on discrimination revealed the very low rate of use of both residential and daycare services by black people in both the mental health and criminal justice systems. The reasons for this are not clear and it is therefore crucial to try to establish at what point in the process black people are dropping out. For example, it may be that they are being referred but not accepted by hostels, but equally they may not be being put forward in the first place. If this is the case, referral agents and not hostel staff need to be the focus of work to improve usage by black people. In reality, this is probably a cumulative process with a drop-out rate at every stage so that all concerned need to review their practices.

Daycare

Referral processes for many forms of daycare are minimalist and there is much to be said for this in terms of informality, acceptance and a clublike sense of voluntarism. With mentally disordered offenders who may pose a threat to staff or others attending a centre, more thought needs to be given to the issue. In particular, fieldwork staff need to be clear about whether they have expectations of the daycentre monitoring the client's behaviour and attendance. If this is the case, then some information needs to be supplied and the client made aware of what is going on. Equally, referral agents need to be mindful of risk. It is dubious practice to use the banner of client confidentiality to justify a referral or request for a service which omits crucial information about dangerousness.

The actual decision to offer a place in a daycentre will depend on many of the considerations outlined in the preceding section on residential admissions. Daycare does offer greater scope for flexibility of approach than residential care because it is not uncommon for individuals to attend on different days depending on what activities are on offer. This means that group mix can be considered on a day-to-day basis and careful planning can allow potentially difficult combinations of clients to be avoided. Care can also be given to ensuring that the client attends groups and activities that match assessed need, rather than a 'job lot' that may be the case when living in a hostel. In theory, a daycentre could operate as a therapeutic community three days a week and as a maintenance and activity base for the other two. Equally, it is possible to have insight-oriented groups running alongside 'depot injection' clinics, though it takes a well-managed and motivated staff group to give equal time and commitment to such different types of professional activities. Miller and Gwynne (1972), when observing units caring for physically disabled people, noted that none were content to be just a repository for the damaged and needy. The same could be said of those providing for the mentally disordered offender group in residential or daycare settings.

THE ETHOS

Residential work

Some hostels explicitly espouse a theory or approach and make it the cornerstone of the daily pattern of living, with staff often attracted by the approach and simultaneously undertaking training that relates to that approach. In the mental health field a good example is the model of the therapeutic community propounded through the Richmond Fellowship by its founder Elly Jansen (1980). Similarly, many alcohol and drug rehabilitation hostels have approaches built around a particular understanding of addiction. It is not the function of this book to review the effectiveness of all such approaches and to come up with a preferred approach for mentally disordered offenders. Nevertheless, the observations made earlier under the heading of Task and Functions still obtain: namely, that the ethos of the hostel should be suited to the assessed needs of the prospective or actual resident. A solely maintenance approach is unlikely to suit an active young person with a personality disorder and a tendency to abuse alcohol or drugs. Some hostels are so explicitly committed to either the horticultural or the maintenance model that it is quite clear whether or not a particular client can fit in with the prevailing ethos. However, many hostels achieve a blend of approaches by insisting that all residents attend certain groups and activities (related to maintenance functions) and only some residents are required to attend groups or individual sessions where growth and change are hoped for and expected. There are, nevertheless, limits to the range of needs that can be met in any one establishment and the wrong mix of residents can undermine even the soundest approach. It also helps team-work and the identity of the staff group if there is a preferred way of working to which all subscribe. This helps to create a positive identity for a unit that can be translated into good publicity material. This in turn should stimulate referrals appropriate to the working method of the unit.

The ethos of a hostel also covers those aspects of its function-ing that may not be conscious or explicit but emerge from the attitudes and values of staff and residents. These relate to what might be termed core values, such as acceptance of the individual, respect for individual choice and a commitment to everyone enjoying as rich an experience of life as circum-stances allow. The latter tends to be indicated by attention to the quality and diversity of food, the decor of the hostel and the comfort of furniture and beds.

Among these unconscious elements that contribute to the ethos of the hostel are unspoken assumptions about race and ethnicity. Many hostels are in reality 'white' hostels, in that the food, pictures and staff are predominantly European. This probably contributes to the low numbers of black people using hostels. To bring about change in this respect will require effort, not just in terms of making equal opportunities policies real by appointing black staff but also by re-evaluating the whole atmosphere of the hostel. Attention will need to be given to whether positive and familiar images of black people are presented on posters and pictures or if such images are either absent, exotic or stereotypical. The involvement and advice of black staff and residents (if any!) is likely to make such a review real rather than tokenistic. Willingness to provide ethnic food as a matter of routine will probably be used as a yard-stick, as this requires thought and planning over time rather than a quick burst of energy and changing the art work!

Consideration should be given to developing an advisory group from local black community groups. They may well be able to provide useful advice on what changes are most critical. It is also possible that such an association will make the hostel more visible and acceptable within the black community and over time this will lead to higher usage by black clients. An alternative is to invite senior members of black community groups to join the management group of the hostel and become involved in issues such as referral sources and admissions. The training manual *Improving Mental Health Practice* produced by the Northern Curriculum Development Group (1993) provides some examples of such initiatives.

Daycare

Much of what has been outlined about the ethos of residential settings also holds good for daycare settings. Certainly such settings are as prone as hostels to be unconsciously Eurocentric and white. The greater use of volunteers in daycare settings does give greater scope for introducing black 'staff' and this should be possible in a short timescale if the trust and co-operation of ethnic minority community groups and leaders can be secured.

The flexibility to run different activities on different days also raises the possibility of identifying certain days when a particular effort will be made to reach out to whichever ethnic minority is most in need in the area. Meals, activities and staff could all be focused on the needs of one cultural group and a truly ethnically sensitive service achieved. Even though this might not be possible on other days, through such a special day the staff will probably become sensitized to cultural issues and this will carry over. For this and other reasons it is important that such initiatives are not left solely to ethnic minority staff to arrange, support and publicize, though their help and advice will be essential. The other main reason for white staff, particularly managers, to be fully involved in any special days is that provision for ethnic minority groups should not be marginalized. If it is, service users will soon pick this up, as will volunteers, and the service may well not be supported. Marginalization also makes for vulnerability and the danger is that when cutbacks are made, such provision will be seen as an optional extra and not as mainstream.

Nick Mounsey (1983) wrote a pithy, helpful article on mental health daycentres called 'It's not what you do it's the way that you do it'. In it he noted a tendency for the planning of such centres to become preoccupied with the details of the daily or weekly programme, with insufficient attention given to the atmosphere or ethos of the whole establishment. To counter this emphasis on detail he took Yalom's eleven curative factors that contribute to the effectiveness of group psychotherapy and used them as a framework for the analysis of process issues in a daycentre (Yalom, 1975). For example, he took one factor like altruism and showed how a day-centre offers opportunities to all those attending to help others and thereby to feel good about themselves. Whether this happens over a cup of tea, at the bus stop or in a group psychotherapy session is not important: it is the oppor-tunity that matters. The right atmosphere may well be more important than the particular approach or philosophy used. This is similar to the finding in the counselling field of the importance of non-specific factors such as warmth, empathy and acceptance.

If this is what might be covered by the term ethos in a daycentre, what if anything needs to be added or taken away for the mentally disordered offender? The necessary element of control and monitoring has been discussed under Task and Purpose, but the question of how to help a member of a doubly stigmatized group has not. The sense of being alone with a unique and terrible problem may be acute for some mentally disordered offenders. There is something to be said for review-ing how such a need can be met. The 'dilution' approach is to take very few referrals of this type and to ensure that numbers never build up to a 'dangerous' level. An alternative is a 'concentration' approach in which part of the programme is adapted particularly for such specialist needs. This allows mentally disordered offenders access to another of Yalom's curative factors, namely universality or the discovery that one's experience is to some extent shared and shareable. To adopt such an approach does require some planning, as preparatory work will be needed. Ideally, a community psychiatric nurse, social worker or probation officer with experience in this field should co-work the group or activity with centre staff or volunteers. It will also be necessary to do some publicity to referral agents to ensure sufficient potential members are available.

DISCHARGE

The prevailing theme of this chapter is the work and planning that needs to be undertaken if residential and day services are to make a positive contribution to community care of the mentally disordered offender. The emphasis has been on what can be achieved if needs are recognized, staff trained and supported, and prejudices and fears acknowledged and worked with. If all this happens, there is a good chance that many more mentally disordered offenders will be able to live in the community with a better rather than a worse quality of life.

It also needs to be recognized that even when such efforts have been made, there is no guarantee that every mentally disordered offender will be able to use the help and support available. Staff in decision-making positions should resist 'over-selling' this group and aim for a realistic rather than an idealistic commitment to care and rehabilitation. If the assessment of risk and monitoring element has been stressed as much as the helping and maintenance functions, then staff may not need too much help in accepting that some people are not progressing and may in fact be deteriorating. It is far better if such a recognition can be made earlier rather than later so that people such as social supervisors are alerted and alternatives such as re-admission to hospital planned. The worst scenario is where the person becomes seriously disordered and a danger to self or others, or commits other types of offences, and has to be arrested or re-admitted to hospital in traumatic and possibly dramatic circumstances.

Much will depend on how the staff group is functioning and the extent to which individuals have identified with a particular resident or client. Work in staff meetings and individual supervision may be needed to enable staff to feel sad and relieved without also having to blame themselves or others for the deterioration in the individual. Ultimately, the duty to society and the individual mentally disordered offender converge because it is in nobody's best interests for anyone to get hurt or be put in danger of being so.

Residential

A discharge from a hostel is unlikely to occur without triggering some sort of official response either from someone with the legal responsibility for supervising the person or for funding the provision, or both. The emphasis is therefore on the way in which this is done. Some of this is covered in the introductory general comments above. A further aspect is to consider that discharge from one place is commonly admission to another, so attention needs to be given to recording and passing on the details of why and how the discharge took place. Whether the next admission is to a hospital or another hostel it is important that information travels with the person, most effectively through a nominated keyworker. If this is not done then very real dangers are likely to emerge. The enquiry into the care and treatment of Christopher Clunis (Ritchie *et al.*, 1994) notes the lack of communication between the various hospitals and workers about his mental health, dangerousness and ability to care for himself. For example, the clinical assistant discharging him from St Charles Hospital told the enquiry that he regarded his patient as 'someone who made a lot of threats with knives and was probably not a dangerous person'. This was despite the fact that during that admission he had stabbed a patient five times!

Residential workers are often reluctant to record events and write reports but this simply cannot be accepted when mentally disordered offenders are involved. Not only may such reluctance lead to others unwittingly being exposed to danger, but it also feeds into the low status of residential work. Professional recognition comes to those who are seen to be competent in doing difficult jobs. Much residential work is necessarily private and may easily escape recognition. Providing written reports for the courts, case conferences and the like is an important part of giving residential workers a voice and thereby gaining recognition. If such efforts are not made, then those best placed to assess the resident are not influencing the decision-making processes. It is not enough to say after the event that 'I told you so' unless that judgement and the evidence for making it have been written down and conveyed to those making the decisions.

Daycare

Discharge from a daycare setting can happen by default when the client simply ceases to attend. In settings which are well staffed, such absences will probably be noted and efforts made to establish the reasons for them. Even so, it is easy for weeks to slip by without making contact with the person. This may be a matter of concern with any person attending a centre but it must be an urgent consideration if the client is a mentally disordered offender who presents a serious risk. Though many find the idea of some sort of 'At Risk' register objectionable, it is now a requirement for national health service provider units and this practice will probably spread to other units that accept mentally disordered offenders. Experience with child protection suggests that such registers can be helpful, as can a requirement for a nominated keyworker and a statutory obligation to hold multiprofessional case conferences. Even where such procedures are in place, there is no substitute for diligence and careful observation. Daycare staff are often well placed in this respect. Fieldwork staff usually see clients in their own homes, at most once a week and possibly not in any interaction with others. Daycare staff, conversely, may see clients two or three times a week, in the centre in inter-action with other staff and clients, so they have a much fuller basis for assessing levels of functioning. Access to this amount of information may be far more significant than the amount of training the worker has had. Untrained staff should therefore be encouraged to voice their observations and concerns, and to communicate these to the keyworker or the head of unit as soon as someone at risk stops attending without good reason.

COMMUNICATION AND PURPOSE IN RESIDENTIAL AND DAYCARE SETTINGS

There have been many references in this chapter to the need for staff to be clear about their task with mentally disordered offenders. There have also been frequent calls for careful monitoring. Both of these depend on good staff communica-tion and teamwork. However, good communication in staff groups is not easily achieved and the reasons for this are partly structural: that is, they rise from the way of working.

Looking first at daycare settings, it is fair to say that most involve a range of activities, with service users commonly having a choice of activities. Different service users may

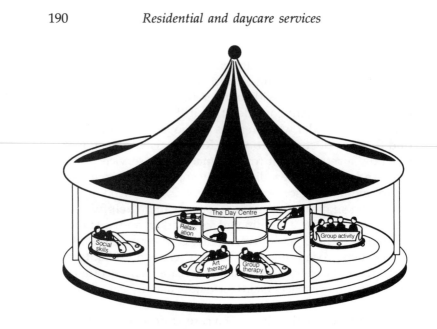

Figure 7.1 The Waltzing Matilda.

attend on each day and some staff may also be sessional or part-time. If we try to conceptualize the activities of a week or even a day it is difficult to hold all the people and groups in our minds. One image is of the fairground ride, The Waltzing Matilda, in which a series of rotating circular open carriages revolve around a central stationary engine and control point. See Figure 7.1, *The Waltzing Matilda*.

Each carriage represents an activity or group meeting. The staff and service users in each group are primarily focused on those in their carriage and they remain with each other for the duration of the ride. They may be dimly aware of what is going on elsewhere but they are not in a position to become involved or to intervene. The only person who can see all the carriages is the centrally placed controller who is also the only person in a stationary position. This may be the head of the daycentre but that person is quite likely to be actually involved in a group meeting or on the telephone. This frequently leaves the receptionist or secretary as a key person in the communication system, something that is often commented on informally but rarely analysed.

The only way that the staff can have a meeting is if the 'ride' stops and the service users are absent. In effect, the only times that the 'ride' is stopped and the staff are present is at the beginning and end of the day. At the end of the day there may be great pressures to catch up on work or go home and it can require a great effort to etablish a pattern of meetings if this has not been the tradition. It is important to have some sort of gathering at the beginning of the day in order to share plans, cover for absent staff and share important information about particular clients. Equally, at the end of the day it is crucial to spend some time together taking stock of developments for both staff and service users. If such meetings do not take place, crucial information may be lost and warning signs missed.

Equally important is the need for regular staff meetings of all the staff who work in a centre. It is difficult to find a time and a day when all can attend and the *Waltzer* is allowed to stop. It is hard for teams to maintain a shared vision of the work and hold to care plans without the opportunity for such meetings. If teams feel they are losing their coherence of vision and shared aims, it may be important to create more time and space for this. 'Away Days' and 'Team Days' can be achieved by closing down the centre for a day or even a week. Such times allow the group to get in touch with what they are trying to achieve and to review the purposes of a centre. Creating such a space might be helpful for a staff group which is contemplating accepting referrals of mentally disordered offenders and needs time to think through the implications of this both individually and as a team.

A third element in maintaining both purpose and communication is leadership. To analyse all the elements of that elusive concept would be far beyond the remit of this chapter. However, it is helpful to consider how a leader can facilitate good communication and provide purpose if they are well positioned in the system. Returning to the fairground analogy, the team leader can get close to staff in a couple of ways. One is to join a particular activity group and work alongside a member of staff. This can be helpful and affirming if the member of staff has asked for such help, though the reverse could be the case if it was experienced as checking up or criticizing. The drawback is that it leaves the rest of the 'Ride'

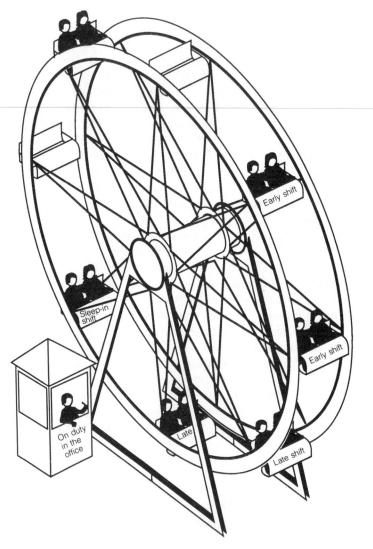

Early shift

Sleep-in shift

Early shift

On duty in the office

Late

Late shift

Figure 7.2 The Big Wheel.

unsupervised and other staff may feel neglected and unsupported. The leader therefore needs to balance time between the central control position and working alongside particular members of staff.

In residential work, the situation is further complicated by the fact that there is commonly activity and staff involvement through 24 hours of the day. Staying with fairground imagery, this can be represented as the *Big Wheel* (Figure 7.2). The seats carry staff and residents and the wheel rotates constantly, pausing only for residents to enter or leave the establishment and for staff to come on and off duty. The challenge is to find ways in which both the staff on duty at the same time (the *Waltzing Matilda* problem) and the staff handing over to the next shift (the *Big Wheel* problem) can communicate well and work with a common purpose. Handover meetings and written communications such as logbooks and diaries are all used to try and address the problems arising from shift working. Full staff meetings are also used but it is not easy to bring everyone together and still perform basic care duties. The *Big Wheel* is generally harder to stop than the *Waltzing Matilda* though this is more possible where residents all attend a daycentre.

Just as in daycare, the leadership function is crucial to a staff team staying on task and in good communication with each other. Given that residential work involves both the *Big Wheel* and the *Waltzing Matilda*, the challenge for the leader to find the right position to lead from is even more problematic. Logic dictates that the leader spends a good deal of time in the control position but this is not a good place to make close relationships with either staff or residents. Once again, the leader has the challenge of blending time in a central management role with time spent alongside others. Finding that blend is difficult but it is essential if residential and daycare settings are to cope well with the challenge of caring for mentally disordered offenders.

SUMMARY

This chapter has treated residential and daycare services separately but under the same four headings of Tasks and Functions, Referrals, Ethos and Discharge. The importance of both services to successful community care has been stressed, as has the need to open up such services to all potential users, especially those from ethnic minority groups. The aim has been to tease out the implications of managing mentally disordered offenders in these settings. Though this may deter some people from taking on this challenge, it is hoped that for others it will provide a helpful structure for planning and working. The chapter ended with a consideration of the very real challenges involved in achieving good teamwork and maintaining a sense of professional purpose in residential and daycare settings.

REFERENCES

Home Office and Department of Health and Social Security (1987) *Mental Health Act 1983 Supervision and After Care of Conditionally Discharged Restricted Patients: Notes for the Guidance of Supervisors,* Home Office, London.

Jansen, E. (ed.) (1980) *The therapeutic community,* Croom Helm, London.

Miller, E. and Gwynne, G.V. (1972) *A Life Apart,* Tavistock, London.

Mounsey, N. (1983) It's not what you do it's the way that you do it. *Community Care,* 20 October, 23–4.

Northern Curriculum Development Project (1993) *Improving Mental Health Practice,* CCETSW, London.

Ritchie, J.H., Dick, D. and Lingham, R., (1994) *The Report of the Inquiry into the Care and Treatment of Christopher Clunis,* presented to the Chairman of North East Thames and South East Thames Regional Health Authorities, HMSO, London.

Smith, G.W. (1993) A view from the Probation Service, in *The Mentally Disordered Offender in an Era of Community Care: New Directions in Provision,* (eds W. Watson and A. Grounds, Cambridge University Press, Cambridge, pp. 18–26.

Yalom, I.D. (1975) *The Theory and Practice of Group Psychotherapy,* Basic Books, New York.

Wiltshire County Council (1988) *Report of a Departmental Inquiry into the Discharge of Responsibilities by the Wiltshire Social Services in Relation to Daniel Mudd from his Release from Broadmoor in May 1983 until his Arrest in December 1986 for the Murder of Ruth Perrett,* Trowbridge, Wiltshire.

8

Key issues for the future

EMERGING CONTRADICTIONS

Mentally disordered offenders, along with the general psychiatric population, have become both beneficiaries and victims of the government's community care policies. They are beneficiaries to the extent that long-term institutional care, along with its accompanying disadvantages, is increasingly being avoided. They are victims to the extent that community facilities, and in some instances community acceptance, has yet to 'catch up' with the reforms.

Over the last 40 years there has been a gradual erosion of secure provision within NHS psychiatric hospitals together with a loss of expertise in managing difficult and potentially dangerous patients. As suitable in-patient facilities have declined in number, there has been an accompanying waning of enthusiasm among staff to care for this group. This is likely to continue with 55 000 mental illness beds in England and Wales in 1991 falling on present trends to just 18 000 by the year 2000. None of these developments have been adequately compensated by the modest growth of beds in the regional secure units. It is not surprising therefore that in this new age of market economics within the health service, a number of private operators have emerged offering highly specialized and secure hospital care. The current market leaders appear to be St Andrews Hospital in Northampton and the services provided by American Medical International Inc at Kneesworth House Hospital and Stockton Hall Hospital.

Interestingly, between 1981 and 1991, while the number of NHS psychiatric beds was contracting, the number of commitments to hospital under Part III of the Mental Health Act 1983 substantially increased. Admissions to special hospitals of restricted patients during this period remained fairly constant and most of the increase was among those admitted to other hospitals (Home Office, 1993). Not surprisingly, some of this increase was absorbed by the private sector. Lee-Evans (1993) reported a clear trend towards a gradual increase in the proportion of detained patients who were involved in criminal proceedings among those admitted to Kneesworth House Hospital and they accounted for 40% of all admissions by 1988/89.

It may be that health authorities and NHS trusts will find it more cost effective to fund extra-contractual referrals to private hospitals than to establish small, expensive, specialized units locally for challenging patients. In any event, it would appear that the current secure private hospitals have exploited a niche in the market and are here for the foreseeable future. Unfortunately, however, their catchment areas cover the whole country and patients will probably be far from their homes and therefore unable to benefit from the locally based service idealized by the community care reforms. Moreover, community-based staff will find liaison more difficult because of the large distances involved.

However, unlike the special hospital, the turnover of patients seems to be fairly swift. Lee-Evans (1993) describes Kneesworth Hospital's primary function as the assessment and treatment of difficult-to-place patients. He feels that, 'the hospital has provided an important refuge for a public sector service at a time of crisis; a short-term placement enables local services either to resolve the crisis situation or to make local arrangements for alternative service provision'. Moreover, there is likely to be considerable pressure on community staff to produce subsequent care plans involving local services fairly quickly, if only to save substantial sums of money when the patient moves out of the private sector and back into the care of district services. Throughcare will probably be a much more active concept and not reserved mainly for the probation service, as has traditionally been the case within the prison system.

The prison system itself is under pressure to reduce the number of mentally ill inmates by transfer to more appropriate psychiatric facilities. Indeed, the growth in the number of 'divert' schemes and panel-assessment schemes means that many fewer mentally disordered petty offenders attract a prison sentence altogether. The result has been that a much greater number of mentally disordered offenders now require care and support in the community than has been the case in previous years. Unfortunately, current mental health legislation is still primarily hospital-based and does not always adequately meet the needs of the patient in the community, nor the community itself.

Disappointingly the limited existing legislation designed to support the mentally ill in the community has been little used. Probation orders with a condition of psychiatric treatment have had a relatively low usage over the years; guardianship orders have been virtually non-existent and the community disposals available under the Criminal Procedure (Insanity and Unfitness to Plead) Act 1991 can be used only for the extremely small number of people found unfit to plead. Section 17 of the Mental Health Act 1983 allows a detained patient's responsible medical officer to sanction up to six months leave in the community while continuing treatment and medication. If the patient fails to comply, he can be recalled from leave by virtue of the original authority. It was previously common practice to recall the patient to hospital at the end of the six months and then extend the order and grant a fresh spell of leave. However, this practice was declared illegal by the High Court in the 1986 Hallstrom case (D of H, 1993a) and brought into focus the paucity of mandatory supervision in the community for needy patients.

Other countries have been less reticent about using community orders for the mentally disordered. Americans, for instance, are inclined to be especially tolerant of gross deviation in behaviour in the community because the assertion of individual freedom of speech and conduct is a basic part of their heritage (Slawson, 1990). Accordingly, detention under US mental health legislation generally requires a demonstration of dangerousness; reasons of health alone are insufficient. However, nearly all American states have some form of community commitment order. In its review of the legal powers on the care of mentally ill people in the community the Department of Health quotes other community order examples in Sweden, Australia and New Zealand (D of H, 1993a).

There was increasing concern in the early 1990s about the growing number of vulnerable mentally ill persons who were slipping through the community care net and a few well-publicized tragedies brought the matter to a head. Notable among these was the case of Christopher Clunis who was suffering from paranoid schizophrenia when he randomly killed Jonathan Zito by stabbing him in the eye on a railway platform on 17 December 1992. This was followed on 31 December 1992 by the televised incident involving Ben Silcock, who had a long history of schizophrenia, being severely mauled after climbing into the lion enclosure at London Zoo. Both cases served to accelerate the review by the Department of Health which culminated in its guidelines on the discharge of vulnerable mentally disordered people and their continuing care in the community (NHS, 1994). The review also resulted in health-authority providers being required to draw up, maintain and use supervision registers for those patients who are most at risk. It also led to proposals to introduce supervised discharged arrangements for non-restricted patients who have been detained in hospital under the Mental Health Act and who present a serious risk to their own health or safety, or the safety of other people, unless their care is supervised.

All these developments have lead to far greater expectations of community-based staff. Patients who were previously cared for in institutional settings are more likely to be supported in the community; patients previously lost to the community care network are increasingly being kept within a supervisory framework. Community staff need to increase their understanding of the needs of mentally disordered offenders and those at risk of becoming mentally disordered offenders, while employing agencies need to extend their support to staff and develop appropriate facilities.

TRAINING

It is likely that the mentally disordered offender will feature far more often on the caseload of community-based staff in the future. It is also fair to assume that many such workers will be inadequately trained and/or experienced for the tasks they have to undertake. As long ago as 1975, Herschel Prins was mourning the loss of specialist mental health skills following the 1972 reorganization of social service departments (Prins, 1975). He found that the situation had been exacerbated by the phasing out of specialist university mental health courses and the inevitable diminution of interest in this area in most generic training. Disappointingly, a recent survey, conducted for the Central Council for Education and Training in Social Work, of probation officers and social workers in 'specialist' settings, found the situation unchanged (Hudson *et al.*, 1993). The report concluded that 'basic training in mental health and forensic topics at DipSW level *for probation officers* is inadquate to meet the demands of main grade work in probation teams'. It also stated that 'other *social workers* taking up employment in the mental health field in the community or hospital settings, are likely to have similar gaps in their basic training'.

The Reed Report (D of H/HO, 1992), also identified shortcomings in the training of fieldwork staff and made recommendations for the improved training of community psychiatric nurses, social workers and probation officers at both qualifying and post-qualifying levels.

CCETSW's review of training for probation officers and social workers (Hudson *et al.*, 1993) is in direct response to recommendations for the same by the Reed Report, and it concludes by making its own recommendations:

Basic training for all students on DipSW courses should cover:

1. risk assessment; personal safety issues;
2. civil rights, equal opportunities and anti-discriminatory practice;
3. recognition of mental disorder and assessment of people who may have mental health problems; and
4. legal issues, including the Mental Health Act 1983 and possibilities for diversion of people with a mental disorder from the criminal justice system.

DipSW training for those planning to specialize in mental health:

The students require:

1. more detailed and practice-oriented material on all four topics listed above;

2. in particular, more detailed knowledge of the Mental Health Act;
3. opportunities to visit forensic settings and prisons, and observe work with mentally disordered offenders; and for some:
4. a placement in a forensic setting.

DipSW training for future probation officers

These students require:

1. more detailed and practice-oriented teaching on the topics listed above, with under the third, some emphasis on the notions of 'personality disorder and 'psychopathy' and of 'treatability', and on the relationship between crime and mental disorder;
2. in relation to the fourth, particular focus on the 'criminal' sections of the Mental Health Act 1983 and on diversion; on the Criminal Procedure (Insanity and Unfitness to Plead) Act 1991 and on relevant sections of the Criminal Justice Act 1991;
3. a placement in a general psychiatric or forensic setting, or failing this, opportunities to visit such settings;
4. opportunities on their probation placement to consider the work of the probation service with mentally disordered offenders, court diversion schemes, etc.

Concurrently with the above recommendations the revised regulations on Approved Social Work training state that adequate emphasis should be given to particular issues relating to mentally disordered offenders and to the working of the criminal justice system. It is suggested that this should include knowledge of supervision provisions of the Criminal Procedure (Insanity and Unfitness to Plead) Act 1991 (CCETSW, 1993).

Specialist training in forensic psychiatry for nurses also appears to be in short supply. Currently the English National Board for Nursing, Midwifery and Health Visiting offer a post-registration award to only two relevant courses: Course 960, Principles of Psychiatric Nursing Within Secure Environments and Course N30, Multi-agency Management of the Mentally Disordered Offender. Course 960 is designed for those working in medium secure units while course N30 is geared more for community staff. The latter course aims to provide ample opportunities for registered nurses, probation officers, social workers, lawyers, police and prison officers to explore and understand the nature of multidisciplinary and multi-agency approaches to care for this group. The course, which is run at Knapsbury Hospital in partnership with the University of Hertfordshire, needs to be replicated in many other parts of the country if community pscyhiatric nurses and other staff are to have an opportunity to adequately prepare for this type of work.

Perhaps of most concern is the situation faced by many other support staff who work in bail hostels, mental health hostels, daycentres, etc. Traditionally, residential and daycare staff have always been undertrained for the often complex task they have to undertake. Often they spend more time in direct one-to-one contact with the client than any other worker. Not only are they often without any formal relevant qual-ifications, they often have little access to more informal training or short courses. This is particularly so for those working in the voluntary sector. If residential and daycare services are to be used safely and productively, placing agencies will have to consider support and training issues. As with all training mentioned there is much scope and need for shared training in order to improve working relationships and partnerships.

MANAGEMENT SUPPORT

There is clear evidence to show that unless they are properly managed and directed, community mental health teams shy away from serving the needs of the people with serious long-term mental disorders (Patmore and Weaver, 1992). Chronic patients are often seen as unattractive to work with, difficult to motivate and not infrequently do not comply with care plans. Understandably, therapeutically inclined mental health professionals prefer to work with more 'rewarding' clients with less intractable problems, who are responsive to intervention. Shepherd (1993) makes the point that mentally disordered offenders are likely to evoke similar negative feelings among mental health workers; managers must take steps to combat this situation. Good support and supervision from experienced high-status practitioners is required to elevate the profile of this work.

Similarly, without sound management support and interest, whole schemes can be jeopardized. In a survey of panel-assessment schemes, the oft-quoted Hertfordshire service had relied mainly on a few individuals who were committed to its operation. Because it was developed with little management support, the lack of clear structured arrangements, roles and responsibilities meant that the scheme faltered whenever key personnel moved on (Hedderman, 1993). This was also seen to be a problem in other areas.

Individuals within the specialist teams can function effectively only with good supervision and support. The more difficult and potentially dangerous the client, the greater the need for adequate agency back-up. Clinical supervision is essential for all workers engaging in face-to-face relationships with an individual in need. The more complex the needs, the greater the demand for skilled supervision. Working with a client who has a history of bizarre and/or murderous tendencies can provoke great anxiety in the worker. Dealing with highly uncertain and ambiguous situations produces much stress and feelings of isolation. It is therefore essential that agencies employ highly skilled and knowledgeable supervisors to provide practice guidance, clear oversight and support.

Supervision in such situations may need to be more searching and confrontational in nature than is customary in other less-demanding therapeutic relationships. Workers may need to be supported in challenging the client and being more probing in their enquiry in order to test the validity of apparent normality. Many workers feel uncomfortable with the intrusive nature of their work, feeling that they always seem to be doubting the client's word. They may need help in avoiding their accepting only the good reports on a client's progress while subconsciously ignoring the warning signs of impending trouble. Good supervision in this context is about helping the worker to face the negatives and supporting difficult decisions and actions.

At a more practical level, senior colleagues continually need to strive to free blockages in communication and foster good relationships in inter-agency working. They should act as facilitators for their staff. Unfortunately, skilled and experienced supervisors in this field are fairly few and far between. Agencies may want to foster other opportunities for such support such as staff support groups with a cross-agency membership. Others may wish to 'buy in' the expertise from private sector services, such as Kneesworth House where the social workers have developed a high level of specialist competence in forensic social work, multidisciplinary teamwork and clinical skills (Hudson *et al.*, 1993). As services for mentally disordered offenders expand, agencies will need to develop clear lines of management responsibility and accountability with an adequate framework of staff support.

JOINT PLANNING AND WORKING

The needs of mentally disordered offenders are complex and well outside the scope of any single agency to cope with. Perhaps more than any other client group where the required service needs to have so many diverse components, effective multi-agency and multiprofessional working is indispensable. Furthermore, statutory services are in themselves insufficient to meet the demand, particularly in relation to residential and daycare. Partnerships with voluntary and independent sector providers will become increasingly necessary in the future, requiring the involvement of non-statutory agencies in both service planning and care planning. It is also increasingly being recognized that families and other informal carers have a part to play in planning services, as do the patients themselves. In any event, patients should always be involved in the planning of their own care programmes.

The requirement for health and local authorities to work together in planning for mental health care services was outlined in the National Health Service and Community Care Act 1990. It directed that effective co-ordinated arrangements be made between health and social service authorities, primary health care teams and voluntary agencies for the continuing health and social care of people with a mental illness, living in their own homes or in residential facilities. This is underlined by the essential requirement for services for mentally disordered offenders which are set out by *The Health of the Nation* (D of H, 1993b). It highlights the need for alliances involving the whole range of relevant agencies to create a better array of services for mentally disordered offenders to help avoid unnecessary imprisonment, with the consequent risk of suicide and self-harm.

However, joint planning is one thing but joint management is quite another. Getting agencies to work together takes skill, patience and time and all these are scarce resources. Joint working creates a different organization, both operationally and managerially, and the more disciplines and agencies involved the more complex the collaboration. Experience of joint agency mental health teams has shown that they are often difficult to manage effectively without clear leadership and direction (Vaughan, 1986).

The model of multidisciplinary working most familiar to people is that of the multidisciplinary hospital team where it

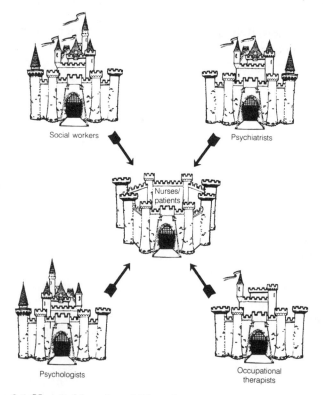

Figure 8.1 Hospital-based multidisciplinary team.

is common for a group of mental health professionals to work together as a team, usually under the leadership of a consultant psychiatrist. Nevertheless, each worker is first and foremost a member of their own professional group or organization, with its own geographical base: social work department, psychology department, etc. The workers leave their base for a common meeting place, usually the hospital ward, and have the patient as their common denominator. Having completed their work together, the staff return or even retreat to their organizational base (Vaughan, 1989), as illustrated by Figure 8.1. Each department has its own hierarchy, procedures, policies, etc., all of which mitigate against effective co-operative practices.

If this model is transferred into the community setting, then joint working becomes extremely difficult and is compounded by the increased number of parties involved when dealing with the mentally disordered offender. All workers need to be

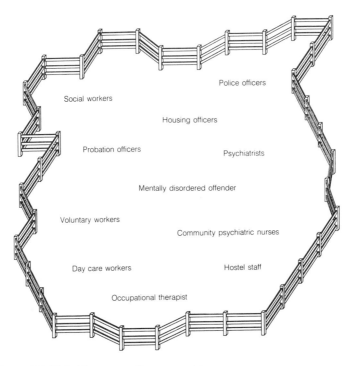

Figure 8.2 Hybrid community support team.

embraced within a common organization framework in order to ensure that a cohesive care plan is followed. Ideally, a hybrid agency needs to be formed where all the relevant personnel can be brought together into one camp, as illustrated in Figure 8.2.

Unfortunately, however, mentally disordered offenders are not a popular group for any of the caring agencies. Local authorities are struggling with limited budgets to meet the needs of politically more attractive customers, such as the elderly and children and families. While striving to focus their attention on those with serious and enduring mental illness, health authorities face opposition from many general practitioners who inundate the community psychiatric service with patients with psycho-neurotic conditions. The criminal justice agencies face growing numbers of 'normal' criminals and an ever-increasing prison population. All agencies are having difficulty in setting priorities and the mentally disordered offender appears to be peripheral to everyone's priorities. It is not surprising that offender patients have been referred to as the people nobody owns' (Prins, 1993). Indeed, Prins goes on to describe them as 'unloved, the unlovely and the unlovable' and as being probably the least attractive to most psychiatric and allied professionals.

Unless there is a strong sense of direction from central government and protection of services against pressure at local level, then this marginalized group will never attract sufficient resources in the community. Funding to local authorities from the Department of Health needs to be ring-fenced in favour of services for mentally disordered offenders in order to ensure that resources are not directed towards competing and more politically attractive priorities at local level. Community care plans prepared by local authorities and health authorities also need to make specific plans and provisions for this group in order to maintain their profile and register their claim on resources. These and other recommendations made by NACRO's Mental Health Advisory Committee (NACRO, 1993) need vigorous pursuit if the needs of the mentally disordered offender are to be met in the future.

REFERENCES

CCETSW (1993) *Requirements and Guidance for the Training of Social Workers to be considered for Approval in England and Wales under the Mental Health Act 1983*, Central Council for Education and Training in Social Work, London.

Department of Health (1993a) *Legal Powers on the Care of Mentally Ill People in the Community*, Report of the Internal Review, Department of Health, London.

Department of Health (1993b) *The Health of the Nation: Key Area Handbook Mental Illness*, HMSO, London.

Department of Health Home Office (1992) *Review of Health and Social Services for Mentally Disordered Offenders and Others Requiring Similar Services*, (Reed Report) Cm2088, HMSO, London.

Hedderman, C. (1993) *Panel Assessment Schemes for Mentally Disordered Offenders*, Research and Planning Unit Paper 76, Home Office, London.

Home Office (1993) *Statistics of Mentally Disordered Offenders England and Wales 1991*, Home Office Statistical Bulletin Issue 92/93, Home Office Research and Statistics Department, Croydon.

Hudson, B.L., Cullen, R. and Roberts, C. (1993) *Training for Work With Mentally Disordered Offenders*, Report of a Study of the Training Needs of Probation Officers and Social Workers, CCETSW, London.

Lee-Evans, M. (1993) A view from the private sector, in W. Watson and A. Grounds (eds) *The Mentally Disordered Offender in an Era of Community Care*, Cambridge University Press, Cambridge, pp. 149–65.

NACRO Mental Health Advisory Committee (1993) *Community Care and Mentally Disturbed Offenders*, Policy paper No. 1, NACRO, London.

National Health Service (1994) *Guidance on the Discharge of Mentally Disordered People and their Continuing Care in the Community*, Health Service Guidelines, HSG (94), 27, London.

Patmore, C. and Weaver, T. (1992) Improving community services for serious mental disorder. *Journal of Mental Health*, 1, 107–15.

Prins, H. (1975) A danger to themselves and to others. *British Journal of Social Work* 5(3), 297–309.

Prins, H. (1993) Offender-patients: the people nobody owns, in W. Watson and A. Grounds (eds) *The Mentally Disordred Offender in an Era of Community Care*, Cambridge University Press, Cambridge, pp. 3–8.

Shepherd, G. (1993) Case management, in W. Watson and A. Grounds (eds) *The Mentally Disordered Offender in an Era of Community Care*, Cambridge University Press, Cambridge, pp. 166–76.

Slawson, P. (1990) Some recent changes to mental health law in the United States, in R. Bluglass and P. Bowden (eds) *Principles and Practice of Forensic Psychiatry*, Churchill Livingstone, Edinburgh, pp. 1217–24.

Vaughan, P.J. (1986) A question of balance. *The Health Service Journal*, 5 September, 1260–1.

Vaughan, P.J. (1989) A new kind of team. *Community Care*, 14 September, 14–15.

Appendix: The Home Office guidelines on social supervision

MENTAL HEALTH ACT 1983

Supervision and after-care of conditionally discharged restricted patients

Notes for the guidance of social supervisors

INTRODUCTION

1. These Notes are for the guidance of social workers or probation officers who take on the role of social supervisor to a patient who, having been made subject to the special restrictions set out in Section 41 of the Mental Health Act 1983 (a restricted patient), is conditionally discharged from hospital by either the Home Secretary or by a Mental Health Review Tribunal under Section 42(2) or 73(2) respectively of the 1983 Act. The term 'social supervisor' is used throughout the Notes to mean the social worker or probation officer who has a responsibility to report to the Home Secretary on the progress in the community of such a patient. The Notes cover the procedures which should take place before the patient leaves hospital, the responsibilities of those involved with the patient after discharge from hospital and the action to be taken in some of the circumstances which may arise while the patient is in the community. The Notes cannot be fully comprehensive and do not represent instructions; much must be left to the discretion of the social supervisor and his or her senior officers. They are intended, however, to cover the broad aspects of the work and to give examples of and guidance in procedures and practices which have been found, over the years, to be most effective.

2. These Notes are issued following a review of procedure and practice in relation to the supervision of conditionally discharged restricted patients which has been carried out by the Home Office in association with the Department of Health and Social Security (DHSS). The review has incorporated discussion with practitioners in the field and in consultation with representative bodies. These Notes replace the previous document, 'Treatment of mentally disordered offenders who are subject to the special restriction set out in Section 41 of the Mental Health Act 1983'. Any questions arising from the Notes, or suggestions for their improvement, should be sent to C3 Division, Home Office, 50 Queen Anne's Gate, London SW1H 9AT. The Notes will be reviewed periodically in the light of comments received.

THE LEGAL AND STATISTICAL FRAMEWORK

Restriction orders and restriction directions

3. Restricted patients represent only a tiny percentage of all patients in mental hospitals. Patients may become subject to restriction orders in one of three ways. (i) Under Section 37 of the Mental Health Act 1983, the court may, where a convicted offender is reported to be suffering from one of the forms of mental disorder defined in that Act, by order authorize his admission to and detention in a hospital for psychiatric treatment. When such an order, known as a hospital order, is made by a Crown court or the Court of Appeal, and it appears that there is a risk of the offender committing further offences if set at large, the court may for the protection of the public from serious harm, make a further order known as a *restriction order*. The principal effect of a restriction order is that the patient may not be allowed leave outside the hospital or be transferred to another hospital without the authority of the Home Secretary, and may not be discharged from hospital except by the Home Secretary or a Mental Health Review Tribunal (see paragraph 7 below).

(ii) Under the Criminal Procedure (Insanity) Act 1964* a person charged with an offence before a Crown Court and found unfit to plead to the charge or not guilty of an offence by reason of insanity must be admitted to a hospital specified by the Home

*Authors' Note: This act has been superceded by the Criminal Procedure (Insanity and Unfitness to Plead) Act 1991.

Secretary and detained there as if he was subject to a hospital order with a restriction order. There are few of these cases each year.

(iii) Under Section 47 of the Mental Health Act 1983, the Home Secretary may make a transfer direction authorizing the transfer to hospital for treatment of mental disorder of a prisoner who is serving a sentence of imprisonment. In doing so he may also make a *restriction direction*, under Section 49 of that Act, which has the same effect, during the patient's detention, as a restriction order but, in the case of a determinate sentence, expires at the end of the sentence. Under Section 48 of that Act the Home Secretary may make a transfer direction on a prisoner who is not serving a sentence of imprisonment – usually one who has been remanded in custody awaiting trial or sentence. A transfer direction under Section 48 almost always carries with it a restriction direction.

4. A restriction order made by a court may be made for a specified period but is usually made without limit of time. The restrictions applying to a patient found unfit to plead or not guilty by reason of insanity are always of indefinite duration. In the case of a transferred prisoner, the restrictions last as long as the sentence of imprisonment imposed or other authority for detention, or until the prisoner is removed back from hospital to prison.

Discharge and recall

5. Under Section 42 of the Mental Health Act 1983, the Home Secretary has the power to bring a restriction order to an end at any time if he is satisfied that it is no longer needed for the protection of the public. This is known as an *absolute discharge*. Under the same Section, the Home Secretary may by warrant discharge a patient subject to conditions at any time while a restriction order is in force. This is known as a *conditional discharge*. The Home Secretary may by warrant recall a conditionally discharged patient and after recall a patient once again becomes subject to detention in hospital with restrictions.

Mental Health Review Tribunals

6. Under the Mental Health Act 1983, a detained restricted patient may apply to have his case heard by a Mental Health Review Tribunal roughly once each year. If he does not apply,

his case will be referred to a Tribunal by the Home Secretary every three years, under Section 71(2). After a conditionally discharged patient has been recalled, the Home Secretary must, under Section 75(1), refer the case to a Tribunal within one month of recall. Under Section 75(2), conditionally discharged patients may apply to a Tribunal once during the second year of their discharge and once in every two-year period thereafter.

7. Prior to the coming into force of the Mental Health Act 1983 on 30 September 1983, Tribunals had no power to make any direction in respect of a restricted patient's case, only to advise the Home Secretary who held exclusive powers of discharge. Since that time, under Section 73 of the Mental Health Act 1983, Tribunals have had the power to discharge a restricted patient absolutely or conditionally providing certain criteria are met. This power does not apply to prisoners who have been transferred to hospital under Sections 47 and 48 of the Mental Health Act 1983 or equivalent earlier legislation. In these cases, under Section 74, Tribunals may only advise the Home Secretary.

8. Where a Tribunal decides to direct the conditional discharge of a patient it may, under Section 73(7), defer that direction until it is satisfied tht adequate arrangements have been made for the discharge to take place. It may impose any conditions on discharge. After a Tribunal has directed the conditional discharge of a patient, the Home Secretary may vary those conditions under Section 73(4). Under Section 75(3), a Tribunal may, on application by a patient conditionally discharged by either a Tribunal or the Home Secretary, vary any condition on discharge, impose fresh conditions or direct an absolute discharge.

9. A Tribunal has no power to direct the recall of a conditionally discharged patient, nor to direct the leave from hospital or the transfer to another hospital of a detained restricted patient.

10. Paragraphs 78 to 84 below deal with the ways in which social supervisors may come into contact with Tribunals and the procedures which apply.

The restricted patient population

11. There are about 1700 restricted patients detained in hospital. Over half are classified as suffering from mental illness, about a quarter from psychopathic disorder and the

remainder from either mental impairment or, most rarely, severe mental impairment. Over 60% hve been convicted of offences of violence against the person, a further 12% of sexual offences and 12% of arson. About 1100 are detained in the special hospitals. There are four special hospitals: Broadmoor, in Berkshire, Rampton, in Nottinghamshire, and Park Lane and Moss Side near Liverpool.* Only patients who require treatment under conditions of special security on account of their dangerous, violent or criminal propensities are admitted to the special hospitals. The special hospitals are managed by the Department of Health directly#, not by the National Health Service. The remaining 600 or so detained restricted patients are scattered among 160 or so National Health Service Hospitals.

12. The number of conditionally discharged patients under active supervision in the community is estimated at 600–700, with supervision divided fairly equally between probation and social services departments.

THE ROLE OF THE HOME OFFICE

13. C3 Division of the Home Office comprises about 30 officers whose sole concern is to carry out the Home Secretary's responsibilities under the Mental Health Act 1983 and related legislation. Among their duties, they arrange for the admission to hospital of patients transferred from prison or under the Criminal Procedure (Insanity) Act 1964; they consider recommendations from responsible medical officers in hospitals for the leave, transfer or discharge of restricted patients, seeking the personal authority or a Home Office Minister in many instances; they prepare documentation for Tribunals hearing restricted patient cases, as required under the Mental Health Review Tribunal Rules 1983; and, after the conditional discharge of a patient by authority of either the Home Secretary or a Tribunal, they monitor the patient's progress and give consideration to the variation of conditions, recall to hospital, or absolute discharge as circumstances require.

14. Staff in C3 Division are not specifically trained in law or in medicine but the Division has wide experience of restricted

---

*Authors' Note: Park Lane and Moss Side have since been amalgamated to become Ashworth Special Hospital.
#They are now managed by the Special Hospitals Service Authority.

patient cases and detailed knowledge of the relevant legislation. C3 staff are ready and willing to discuss the case of any
restricted patients with a social supervisor or with his or
her senior officer. Such discussions may be useful for the
exchange of information or simply the sharing of experiences
or problems.

15. In C3 Division, officers of different grades form teams,
each of which deal with work relating to a proportion of the
restriction patient population. The population is divided
alphabetically, according to the patient's surname initial.
Written communications should be addressed, where possible,
to a named officer. The letter to the social supervisor which
accompanies these Notes in an individual case should contain
a name and a telephone number for use in that case. If it does
not, or if in any doubt, a supervising officer wishing to make
telephone contact should telephone 071-273 3000 and ask
to speak to an officer in C3 Division Mental Health Section
dealing with the case of Mr/Mrs/Miss ——. Arrangements for
making urgent telphone contact out of office hours are given
in paragraph 61 below.

THE PURPOSE OF CONDITIONAL DISCHARGE

16. The Home Secretary will usually decide to make a
restricted patient's discharge from hospital subject to certain
conditions. The conditions usually imposed by the Home
Secretary are those of residence at a stated address, supervision by a local authority social worker or a probation officer
and psychiatric supervision. Tribunals also are likely to make
discharge directions conditional either for the protection of the
public or of the patient himself, and to impose similar conditions. If they do not, the Home Office, under Section 73(4)
of the Mental Health Act 1983, usually requires social and
psychiatric supervision.

17. The purpose of the formal supervision resulting from
conditional discharge is to protect the public from further
serious harm in two ways: first, by assisting the patient's
successful reintegration into the community after what may
have been a long period of detention in hospital under conditions of security: second, by close monitoring of the patient's
progress so that, in the event of subsequent deterioration in
the patient's mental health or of a perceived increase in the
risk of danger to the public, steps can be taken to assist the
patient and protect the public. Conditional discharge also

allows a period of assessment of the patient in the community before a final decision is taken whether to remove the control imposed by the restriction order by means of an absolute discharge.

PRE-DISCHARGE PROCEDURES

PREPARATION OF SUPERVISION AND AFTER-CARE

Arrangements by the discharging hospital

On admission of a restricted patient to hospital, the responsible medical officer (the consultant psychiatrist in charge of the case) will, together with the rest of the multidisciplinary clinical team, seek not only to treat the patient's mental disorder but to understand the relationship, if any, between the disorder and the patient's behaviour. The aim will be to understand what led to the dangerous behaviour which resulted in the patient's detention and, as the mental disorder is treated in hospital, to assess the extent to which that treatment is likely to reduce the risk of the patient behaving in a dangerous manner if returned to the community. In some cases this period of assessment and treatment may take several years. Only when the patient's condition has so improved that the level of risk to the public is reduced to the extent that detention in hospital is no longer considered to be necessary, will the clinical team consider recommending the patient's conditional discharge.

19. Staff in the detaining hospital will begin preparations for a patient's conditional discharge before authority for discharge is sought. These preparations include the patient's personal preparation for life outside the hospital and the consideration and choice of suitable accommodation, employment or other daytime occupation, a social supervisor and a supervising consultant psychiatrist.

20. Separate guidance is issued to hospitals about the importance of careful preparation of the arrangements for the supervision and after-care of a patient. A checklist of the main points of that guidance is at Annex C to these Notes. In some cases contact may have been maintained between the patient and his social worker or probation officer during the patient's stay in hospital (and this is to be encouraged). In other cases hospital staff are advised that as soon as the prospective social supervisor and the prospective supervising psychiatrist are

known, they should be involved in discussion of the patient's after-care and supervision arrangements. These discussions are important both as a means of combining hospital and community expertise in the setting up of practical arrangements most suited to the patient and also in enabling the prospective supervisors to familiarize themselves with the patient before discharge.

21. Wherever possible, pre-discharge contact should include at least two visits to the hospital by the social supervisor to meet the patient and participation in at least one multi-disciplinary case conference at which the prospective social supervisor can discuss the case and the plans for discharge with the responsible medical officer, the hospital social worker, the nursing staff who know the patient well, any other hospital staff who have been involved and the prospective supervising psychiatrist. If a social supervisor is asked to take on the case of a restricted patient shortly to be conditionally discharged and is not invited by the hospital to participate in pre-discharge discussion in this way, he or she should request contact with the hospital clinical team through the responsible medical officer, the hospital social worker or the liaison probation officer where one exists. C3 Division of the Home Office may be able to help in cases of difficulty.

CHOICE OF SOCIAL SUPERVISOR

22. Both the social services departments, with experience of assisting clients with a wide range of social difficulties, control of a variety of community resources and a framework for liaison with the Health Service, and the probation service, with wide experience in statutory supervision of clients with a background of offending, are well-qualified to fulfil the role of social supervisor. Both agencies have a statutory basis for doing so: the probation service under the Probation Rules and the social services departments under the general duty expressed in Section 117 of the Mental Health Act 1983. In an individual case the choice of a social supervisor will be made with the particular needs of the patient in mind.

23. Whether a social worker or a probation officer becomes a social supervisor in any particular case will depend on a number of factors. The responsible medical officer and the clinical team may consider, having regard to the patient's history, mental state and likely requirements in the community that one or the other agency is better placed to undertake

the task. The wishes of the patient may also be a relevant, though not determining factor. The patient may have been supervised by one of the other agencies prior to his admission to hospital, and in some cases there may have been ongoing contact with one of the supervising agencies during the patient's stay in hospital which would indicate the appropriate agency for supervision after discharge. In these cases, the hospital social work department will write to the Director of Social Services or Chief Probation Officer as appropriate, giving background information about the patient and seeking the nomination of a social supervisor. In some cases, however, although the clinical team knows what kind of social supervisor a particular patient needs, it may not be known which agency can best meet those needs. In cases which are not clearcut, it is important that both agencies in the local area should have an opportunity to contribute to the decision whether supervision should be provided by a social worker or a probation officer.

24. Except in clearcut cases, discharging hospitals are advised to contact the Director of Social Services for the area to which the patient is likely to be discharged and the appropriate Chief Probation Officer informing them of the likely discharge of a patient and inviting both agencies to meet with the hospital social work department to discuss the selection of a social supervisor. The letter should give information about the patient's social history, criminal history, history of mental disorder and after-care and supervision needs, and should give any views on the type of supervision required.

PROVISION OF WRITTEN INFORMATION BY THE DISCHARGING HOSPITAL

25. In addition to the pre-discharge contact recommended in paragraphs 21 and 24 above, it is essential that the social supervisor should receive, as early as possible before discharge, detailed written information about the patient which can be retained for reference in the files of the supervising agency. Thus, when a social supervisor moves on, the incoming supervisor has access to full written information about the case, as do senior officers in the agency at any time. (In the case of probation supervision, copies of written information will be sent to both the Chief Probation Officer and the nominated supervisor.)

26. Discharging hospitals are advised that the full information provided to the social supervisor for retention should cover the following aspects of the case:

a) a pen-picture of the patient including his diagnosis and current mental state;
b) admission social and medical history;
c) summary of progress in hospital;
d) present medication and reported effects and any side-effects;
e) any warning signs which might indicate a relapse of his mental state or a repetition of offending behaviour together with the time lapse in which this could occur;
f) a report on present home circumstances; and
g) supervision and after-care arrangements which the hospital considers appropriate and inappropriate in the particular case.

If a social supervisor has not received the information detailed before the date of discharge, it should be requested from the discharging hospital. If such a request is not met, it should be notified, in the last resort, to C3 Division of the Home Office.
27. In addition, the discharging hospital may provide details of the circumstances of the offence which led to the patient's admission to hospital and of the legal authority for that admission. As a matter of course, however, this information, together with a note of any relevant previous convictions, will be provided directly by the Home Office as soon as the name of the social supervisor is known. If this information is not received, C3 Division should be notified.

POST DISCHARGE PROCEDURES

MANNER AND FREQUENCY OF SUPERVISION

28. It is the Home Secretary's hope that, by means of conditional discharge of a restricted patient, a situation of danger to the patient or to others can be averted by effective supervision, by appropriate support in the community or by recall to hospital if need be. He recognizes that this hope places great reliance on the personal skills and dedication of individual social supervision. While it will not always be possible to predict and thus prevent dangerous behaviour, it is important that the social supervisor sets out to provide more than just crisis intervention.

29. The specific requirements of supervision will vary from case to case and an individual patient's needs will vary over time. It is impossible, therefore, to draw up a blueprint for successful supervision. However, there are some elements in the role of a social supervisor which are important if supervision is to be effective in achieving its purpose.

30. A social supervisor will have many difficult decisions to make when working with a conditionally discharged patient. The patient should consult the supervisor when considering any significant change in circumstances, for example, a new job, a new home, financial matters or a holiday. Careful consideration of risk should precede any such proposal and the supervisor should advise the patient against taking any step which, in the supervisor's view, would involve an unacceptable degree of risk. Some proposals will involve the social supervisor making a special report to the Home Office (see references to change of address and holidays in paragraphs 54 and 56 below). In accordance with normal practice, probation officers should share the responsibility for difficult decisions concerning conditionally discharged patients with senior officers and Assistant Chief Probation Officers.

31. A sound knowledge of the case is essential if the social supervisor is to be able to spot warning signs before dangerous behaviour occurs. Section 5 above recommends that before discharge the supervising officer should have an opportunity to discuss the patient with those in hospital who know him best. Section 7 covers the provision of written information by the hospital to the supervision officer including specifically, any known warning signs. Social supervisors should seek to build on this initial background to the case by establishing a close relationship with the patient after discharge. In a close relationship, changes in the patient's mental state, behaviour or circumstances are likely to be reported to or noticed by the supervisor. If the patient is in close contact with, or living with, friends or relatives, the social supervisor should also see them regularly.

32. The protection of the public from serious harm is best assured, in the long run, by the sucessful reintegration into the community of the patient. Supervisors should therefore have a positive and constructive approach towards the patient's social rehabilitation rather than simply monitoring progress. Focusing on some positive future achievable goal, rather than measuring success by an absence of failure, is more likely to succeed.

33. Close supervision is important, but this cannot be assured by any set prescription for the nature or frequency of meetings with the patient. Every effort should be made to build a working relationship with the patient. He may resent the continuing control of his life imposed by a conditional discharge and fear the 'policing' role of the supervisor.

34. There is a certain level of supervision which should be maintained if possible changes in a patient's mental state or behaviour are quickly to be spotted. It is recommended that meetings should take place at least once each week for at least the first month after discharge, reducing to once each fortnight and then once each month as the social supervisor judges appropriate. These are considered to be minimum periods. Sometimes the Home Office will request more frequent meetings take place. Generally, individual supervisors will consider more frequent meetings appropriate, particularly for the initial period of the first year during which the patient settles down to life in the community. Meetings should usually take place on the patient's home territory but some meetings away from the home, perhaps in the supervisor's office, may also prove valuable. If, after some time, a social supervisor considers that supervision at monthly intervals is unduly frequent, then he should consider the case for recommending discharge from conditions, having read section 14 below on the length of supervision and absolute discharge.

35. When a social supervisor is absent from their post even for a short period, for example when on leave, it is important that responsibility for the case should be transferred to a colleague and that both the patient and the supervising psychiatrist should know whom to contact as social supervisor. If absences are to be for longer than two months, the Home Office should also be informed. Paragraph 55 below deals with permanent changes of social supervisor.

36. When changes in social supervisors occur, it is important that the outgoing supervisor passes to his successor full information about the case and supplements this with an oral briefing. A change of supervisor may be upsetting for a patient and care should be taken to ease the transition.

37. As well as the importance of a close and informed relationship between the supervising officer and the patient, the most valuable element in successful supervision is liaison with other professionals involved in the case. This aspect is discussed separately in the section on liaison with others involved in the patient's care.

DISCLOSURE OF INFORMATION

38. There can be no hard and fast rules about the nature of information to be disclosed and to whom. Both the social supervisor and the supervising psychiatrist will have detailed information about the patient's case. However, many other people may become involved with the patient in the community and the supervisors will need to consider whether certain information about the patient should be disclosed to such people. Except where medical information is concerned, it will usually be the social supervisor who has to make such decisions. Those to whom it may be appropriate to disclose information about a patient's background include hostel staff, landladies or landlords, employers, those providing voluntary work and, in some circumstances, girlfriends or boyfriends.

39. Decisions about disclosure of information should be taken by social supervisors in the light of their knowledge of the case and their professional judgement and in cases of doubt they will almost certainly find consultations with their line managers helpful. In general, information about the patient should be disclosed only with the full knowledge and agreement of the patient and information should only be given against the patient's wishes when there are strong overriding reasons for doing so. Such reasons may include the patient's known propensity for offending in circumstances to which the accommodation or job may give rise. For example, the supervisor of a patient with a history of offending against a child should be particularly conscious of that fact in discussion with those providing accommodation which does or may also contain children or those providing employment or voluntary work which may bring the patient into contact with children.

LIAISON WITH OTHERS INVOLVED IN THE PATIENT'S CARE

The supervising psychiatrist

40. The consultant psychiatrist who acts as the supervising psychiatrist to a conditionally discharged patient is responsible for all matters relating to the mental health of the patient. The manner in which that responsibility is carried out in a case will depend on the needs of the patient. However, the psychiatrist, like the social supervisor, is asked to report to the Home Office on the patient's condition one month after discharge and

every three months thereafter. (A brief summary of the guidance issued to supervising psychiatrists is at Annex B.)

41. Where the patient requires medication for the treatment of mental disorder after leaving hospital, the supervising psychiatrist will be responsible for making the arrangements for the administration of any necessary medication and for monitoring its effects. (See also the reference in paragraph 46 below to general practitioners.)

42. Should the patient's mental health deteriorate, the supervising psychiatrist will consider whether steps are necessary to arrange for the patient to receive additional out-patient treatment or to be admitted to hospital for treatment, whether voluntarily, under civil powers or by recall (see also the section below on action in the event of concern about the patient's condition). Any decision to admit the patient for short-term treatment, either on a voluntary basis or under civil powers of detention, will generally be taken with the knowledge of and often in consultation with the social supervisor, and in all cases he should be advised when the patient is admitted or discharged in these circumstances.

43. Close liaison with the supervising psychiatrist is essential if supervision is to be effective. Both suprvisors should be involved in the pre-discharge discussions about the patient's after-care and it is expected that they will meet at least once at this stage. They should agree a common overall approach to the patient's treatment, after-care and reintegration into the community and discuss how they can liaise effectively after discharge.

44. If the patient will be taking medication, the supervising psychiatrist should inform the general practitioner and the social supervisor of the nature of the medication, its effects on the patient's condition and behaviour and any possible side-effects. The psychiatrist should also inform the social supervisor of the arrangements to be made for the medication to be given, including when, where and by whom, and of any changes in those arrangements. With this information the social supervisor, while not primarily concerned with the patient's mental health, may identify aspects of the patient's state of mind during his or her regular contact with the patient which might be helpful to the psychiatrist.

45. The social supervisor should send a copy of all reports to the Home Office to the supervising psychiatrist. Similarly, the supervising psychiatrist is advised to send a copy to the

social supervisor of his reports to the Home Office. If these exchanges do not take place, C3 Division should be notified.

Other professionals

46. All conditionally discharged patients should be registered with a general medical practitioner and arrangements for this should be made by the discharging hospital. The supervising psychiatrist and the social supervisor should always bear in mind the need to keep the general practitioner informed of any significant development in this case.

47. Other clinical staff involved may include a community psychiatric nurse or a psychiatric nurse based at the supervising psychiatrist's hospital whose responsibilities would include visiting the patient to administer or monitor his medication.

48. Finally, hostels and centres providing daycare are likely to have several members of staff involved with the patient on a day-to-day basis.

49. The social supervisor will usually be the key worker in liaison between those involved in the patient's care and support. At the beginning of supervision and with subsequent changes in arrangements, the social supervisor should discuss the broad approach to the patient's after-care with others involved and invite them to contact him or her if there is any cause for concern about the patient's condition or behaviour.

REPORTS TO THE HOME OFFICE

50. The Home Office usually asks for reports on the patient's progress from both supervisors one month after conditional discharge and every three months thereafter. Reports are submitted to the Home Office whether the patient was discharged by authority of the Home Secretary or by direction of a Tribunal. In some cases, the Home Office may ask for more frequent reports in the initial period after discharge. This would be made clear at the beginning of supervision. If a report is not received at the required time, a reminder is sent.

51. After a period in the community when a conditionally discharged patient has settled down and is maintaining a steady pattern of life, the social supervisor may consider it appropriate to submit reports to the Home Office at longer intervals. If this decision reflects a belief that the patient can

manage well without active supervision, the supervisor should, in consultation with the supervising psychiatrist, consider whether a recommendation should be put forward to the Home Office for the patient's absolute discharge (see the section below on length of supervision and absolute discharge). If, however, the patient continues to require some formal supervision, the social supervisor may write to the Home Office recommending that his or her reports be made at six-monthly intervals. The Home Office will not agree to reporting intervals of more than six months while supervision continues.

52. It is helpful if reports to the Home Office are completed in the manner shown on the sample form attached to these Notes at Annex A. After the completion of initial summary data, the report itself should convey sufficient information to enable the Home Office to consider whether the patient may remain in the community or whether, in the patient's own interests or for the protection of the public, steps should be taken to return him to hospital. The report should include a detailed account of the patient's current circumstances including accommodation, employment, training, major relationships and other interests and spare-time activities, any changes since the previous report and the reasons for those changes. Reference should be made to any notable improvements or achievements by the patient. If the social supervisor has identified any signs of deterioration in the patient's mental health or behaviour, these should be described in detail, together with any steps already taken to improve the situation and any further proposals for doing so. Finally, the report should include the social supervisor's plans for the patient's continued rehabilitation.

53. All reports to the Home Office should be copied to the supervising psychiatrist and discussed with them as necessary. For one year following discharge, two copies of each report should also be sent, for information, to the responsible medical officer in the hospital which discharged the patient (if the responsible medical officer is not also the supervising psychiatrist).

Changes in address or social supervisor

54. The warrant or direction for the patient's conditional discharge, of which the social supervisor should have a copy usually specifies a named address at which the patient must reside. If the patient wishes to change his address or to be

away from that address for more than a short absence, and the social supervisor agrees that the new accommodation proposed is suitable, the supervisor should write to C3 Division of the Home Office to seek agreement to a change in the condition attaching to discharge (although in an emergency the social supervisor may have to agree to a change of address without prior reference to the Home Office, in which case he should contact C3 as soon as possible afterwards). Agreement to routine changes of address may be sought at any time before the proposed change and need not await the next quarterly report. It would be helpful if details were given of the new accommodation proposed and the reasons for the change. In agreeing to a change the Home Office will issue a formal amendment to the warrant of discharge. The supervising psychiatrist should also be informed (see paragraph 57 below).

55. Although the names of supervisors are not usually entered on a warrant of discharge it would be helpful if the Home Office was notified as soon as there is a permanent change of social supervisor. (Paragraph 35 above deals with temporary absences from work of the social supervisor, for example during leave.)

Patient's holidays

56. A conditionally discharged patient is not precluded by his status from having holidays away from home. The patient should always discuss plans for such holidays with the social supervisor so that the suitability of the arrangements can be considered. During the first six months after discharge, absences from home of more than a few days are not usually advisable. If the patient is to be away for two weeks or more the social supervisor should notify the social services department or probation service (as appropriate) in the holiday area and should inform the patient whom to contact there in case any problems arise. Holidays abroad do not allow any form of supervision to continue and should be considered carefully. Any proposals for the patient to leave the United Kingdom should be put to the Home Office for approval.

57. The supervising psychiatrist should be informed of any of the above proposals. In the case of proposed absences from the patient's home, consideration of special medication arrangements to cover the absence may be necessary.

POST-DISCHARGE CONTACT WITH THE DISCHARGING HOSPITAL

58. The practice of copying supervisor's reports to the discharging hospital for a period of about one year after discharge is intended to produce a number of benefits. For supervisors the sharing of community experience of the patient with the discharging hospital can prepare the way for potentially valuable contact with staff there. A social supervisor who needs further background information about a patient or to discuss the patient's behaviour should make direct contact with the hospital social work department. Most hospitals will expect and welcome such approaches.

ACTION IN THE EVENT OF CONCERN ABOUT THE PATIENT'S CONDITION

59. If a social supervisor is concerned about a conditionally discharged patient's mental state or behaviour, the concern should first be discussed, if possible, with the other professionals involved in the case, particularly the supervising psychiatrist.

60. If the social supervisor has reason to fear for the safety of the patient or of others, he should contact the supervising psychiatrist immediately. The consultant may decide to initiate local action to admit the patient to hospital without delay, either with the patient's consent or using civil powers such as those under Sections 2, 3 or 4 of the Mental Health Act 1983. Whether or not such action is taken, and even if the supervising psychiatrist does not share the social supervisor's concern, the social supervisor should report to the Home Office at once so that consideration should be given to the patient's formal recall to hospital. In accordance with normal practice, recommendations by probation officer supervisors for consideration of recall should be accompanied by the views of a senior probation officer and of the Chief Probation Officer, where this is possible, without undue delay.

61. Telephone discussion in such circumstances is welcomed by staff in C3 Division at the Home Office. In normal office hours an officer on one of the following numbers should be contacted at the Home Office, 50 Queen Anne's Gate, London SW1H 9AT, depending on the surname initial of the patient:

A–D   071 273 3233   (currently Miss H. KcKinnon)
E–J   071 273 2229   (currently Mr W. Dyce)

K–P   071 273 3021   (currently Mr N. Jordan)
Q–Z   071 273 2654   (currently Mr L.H. Hughes)

or ask the switchboard on 071 273 3000 for an officer in C3 Division Mental Health Section.

Outside office hours the duty officer at the Home Office should be contacted, on 071 213 3611, who will in turn contact a member of C3 Division staff at home. A telephone report should be followed up by a written report as soon as practicable.

Recall

62. It is not possible to specify all the circumstances in which the Home Secretary may decide to exercise his powers under Section 42(3) of the Mental Health Act and to recall to hospital a conditionally discharged patient, but in considering the recall of a patient he will always have regard to the safety of the public. A report to the Home Office should always be made in a case in which:

a)   there appears to be an actual or potential risk to the public;
b)   contact with the patient is lost or the patient is unwilling to co-operate with supervision;
c)   the patient's behaviour or condition suggests a need for further inpatient treatment in hospital;
d)   the patient is discharged with or convicted of an offence.

63. Consideration of a case for recall will take into account any steps taken locally to remove the patient from the situation in which he presents a danger. The Home Secretary would have no objection to a conditionally discharged patient being admitted to a hospital, either informally or using the civil powers mentioned in paragraph 60 above, for a short period of observation or treatment but the Home Office and the social supervisor should be kept informed in these circumstances since the patient will again be subject to the formal condition of his earlier discharge when he leaves hospital. However, it is generally inappropriate for a conditionally discharged patient to remain in hospital for more than a short time informally or under civil power of detention, and the Home Secretary would usually wish to consider the issue of a warrant of recall if the period of in-patient treatment seems likely to be protracted.
64. In cases where it seems that admission is necessary to protect the public from possible harm, the supervising

psychiatrist may recommend that the patient be formally recalled to a hospital. The Home Secretary would normally be prepared to act on such a recommendation.

65. Whether the Home Secretary decides to recall a patient depends largely on the degree of danger which the particular patient might present. Where the patient has in the past shown himself capable of serious violence, comparatively minor irregularities in behaviour or failure of co-operation would be sufficient to raise the question of the possible need for recall. On the other hand, if the patient's history does not suggest that he is likely to present a serious risk, the Home Secretary may not wish to take the initiative unless there are indications of a probable physical danger to other persons. There are cases in which recall to hospital for a period of observation can be seen as a necessary step in continuing psychiatric treatment. There are other cases in which antisocial behaviour may be unconnected with mental disorder, so that recall to hospital is not an appropriate sanction and there may be no alternative to leaving the conditionally discharged patient to be dealt with as necesssary by the normal processes under the criminal law. Each case is assessed on its merits in the Home Office and a decision is reached after consultation with the doctor(s) concerned and with the social supervisor.

66. Where recall is considered by the Home Secretary to be necessary and a warrant is signed to that effect, the patient may be returned in the most appropriate manner to the hospital specified on the warrant. If the patient will not return to hospital willingly, on being told of his recall, then the police, to whom a copy of the warrant will have been sent, should be informed. There is generally a duty to inform the patient at the time of his recall of the reasons for that recall. Where a social supervisor is involved in returning the patient to hospital, this duty should be borne in mind. C3 Division should be informed as soon as a recalled patient is back in hospital, or in case of any difficulty.

67. After recall a patient is once again detained as a restricted patient in pursuance of the legal authority which was operating immediately before the conditional discharge. In some cases, the patient may need to return to hospital for only a short while, but in others, the lessons learned in the community may point to the need for a longer stay in hospital. The Home Secretary is obliged to refer the cases of a recalled patient to a Tribunal within one month of recall. The social supervisor and the supervising psychiatrist will become involved in those Tribunal

proceedings and paragraphs 78 to 84 give guidance in such circumstances.

Absconding patients

68. A conditionally discharged patient may leave the approved address and break off contact with both supervisors. In such cases, the social supervisor should report the fact to the Home Office immediately and then make every reasonable effort to locate the patient, contacting his colleagues in other areas if he has reason to believe that the patient may have gone to a particular place in a different locality. The Home Office may simply decide to wait until the patient's whereabouts are known. If necessary, however, the Home Secretary will issue a warrant for the recall of the patient, thus providing the police with the powers to bring the patient into custody.

69. If a conditionally discharged patient is suspected of having left his approved address to go abroad, the Home Secretary may decide to issue a recall warrant and alert the immigration authorities who would detain the patient on re-entry to the country.

Further offending

70. If a conditionally discharged patient has committed an offence and legal proceedings are pending, the Home Secretary will usually consider it advisable, if the patient is in safe custody and presents no danger to others, to let the law take its course so that the court may reach a fresh decision on the need for medical treatment or other measures, rather than recall the patient to hospital. The patient, however, may be recalled if that is in agreement with the court's wishes and the doctor concerned agrees (for example, if the court decides, on conviction, to take no action or to impose a nominal penalty in the knowledge that the patient will be returned at once to hospital).

71. If a conditionally discharged patient is convicted of a further offence and the court imposes a non-custodial sentence, the terms of the previous conditional discharge will continue and the supervisors should resume their roles.

72. If a conditionally discharged patient is convicted of a further offence and the court imposes a sentence of imprison-

ment, the Home Secretary will usually decide to reserve judgement on the patient's status under the Mental Health Act 1983 until he nears the end of his prison sentence. At that stage, the Home Secretary will decide whether to authorize the patient's absolute discharge from liability under that Act, to allow his continued conditional discharge under conditions of residence, social supervision and psychiatric supervision or to direct his recall to hospital on release from prison. Which decision is taken will largely depend on the length of the prison sentence imposed, the nature of the offence, the patient's mental state, both at the time of the offence and during the sentence of imprisonment, and the risk of danger to the public.

LENGTH OF SUPERVISION AND ABSOLUTE DISCHARGE

73. Where a conditionally discharged patient is subject to a restriction order of specified duration, then on the date of expiration of the order he is automatically absolutely discharged from liability to conditions or to be recalled.

74. Where, as in most cases, the restriction order is of indefinite duration, the Home Secretary normally requires active supervision and reporting to be kept up for at least five years after discharge in serious cases, and for at least two years in less serious ones. In some cases, for example, where a patient requires continued medication in the community for the control of symptoms which might otherwise lead to violent behaviour, it may be necessary to retain conditions for a much longer period.

75. If a social supervisor considers that the patient no longer requires active supervision and that the safety of the public would not be at risk if the patient were not subject to such supervision, the matter should be discussed with the supervising psychiatrist before an appropriate recommendation is put forward to the Home Office. The Home Secretary will wish to see evidence of a prolonged period of stability in the community which has been tested by a variety of normal pressures or experiences and it is unlikely that he will be satisfied after periods much shorter than those mentioned above. However, supervisors should use their judgement and put forward a recommendation for an end to formal supervision whenever they consider it appropriate.

76. When the Home Secretary agrees to the absolute discharge of a conditionally discharged patient, a warrant will be

issued and copied to both the patient and the supervisors. Such a decision does not, of course, preclude continuing contact between the patient and the supervisors on a non-statutory basis.

77. As noted in paragraph 8 above, Mental Health Review Tribunals have the power to hear the case of a conditionally discharged patient and either to direct a variation in the conditions attaching to discharge or to direct absolute discharge. In either case, the Tribunal itself will notify the patient and the Home Office, who, in turn, will then write to both supervisors informing them of the decision. In cases of probation supervision, the Chief Probation Officer will also be informed.

MENTAL HEALTH REVIEW TRIBUNALS

78. As paragraphs 6–10 above suggest, there are two circumstances in which a social supervisor may become involved with a Mental Health Review Tribunal. First, when a conditionally discharged patient applied to a Tribunal to have his case heard under section 75(3) of the Mental Health Act 1983, is for variation of conditions or absolute discharge. Second, when the case of a conditionally discharged patient who has been recalled to hospital is referred to a Tribunal under Section 75(1) of that Act. This section of the Notes deals with the procedures likely to affect social supervisors in those circumstances.

79. Mental Health Review Tribunals are held in informal conditions. For restricted patients they are chaired by a Judge and also comprise a psychiatrist and a lay member. All administrative Tribunal business is handled by the Tribunal Clerks' offices, and supervisors should address any general queries about a patient's Tribunal to the appropriate regional office.

Conditionally discharged patients' Tribunals

80. When a conditionally discharged patient applies to a Tribunal, the Tribunal will ask the Home Office to provide a statement containing the information specified in Parts C and D of Schedule 1 to the Mental Health Review Tribunal Rules 1983. This information inclues a report from a supervising psychiatrist on the patient's medical history and presents his

mental condition and a report from the social supervisor on the patient's progress in the community since discharge from hospital.

81. On receipt of the Tribunal's request the Home Office will write to the social supervisor asking for a report, including details of the patient's home circumstances, response to supervision and general progress, and the supervisor's views on the value of continuing social supervision. The supervisor will be asked to reply to the Home Office within four weeks and it is important that this deadline is met. The Tribunal Rules (Rules 6 and 12) provide that the Home Office statement, including the supervisor's reports, will be disclosed to the patient in full unless the Home Secretary recommends, and the Tribunal agrees that part of it, submitted separately, is witheld from the patient. The social supervisor should consider whether his or her report to the Home Office can be fully disclosed to the patient. If not, the part not suitable for disclosure should be recorded on a separate sheet of paper, and the reasons for its non-disclosure explained.

82. The supervisor will not necessarily be informed by the Tribunal of the date of the Tribunal hearing or invited to appear at the hearing, but they may be. In some cases the patient may ask a supervisor to speak on his behalf and in others the Tribunal may call a supervisor to appear.

83. The Tribunal's decision in the case of a conditionally discharged patient is notified to the Home Office, who will inform the supervisors of the nature of the decision.

Recalled patients' Tribunals

84. When a recalled patient's case is referred to a Tribunal or such a patient applies in his own right, statements will be prepared for the Tribunal both by the hospital to which the patient is recalled and by the Home Secretay. The Home Secretary's statement will be concerned primarily to give an account of the circumstances which led to the recall and to give views on whether the patient is yet fit again to be discharged. In referring to the decision to recall, the Home Secretary is likely to draw on reports received from supervisors. In some cases the Tribunal may decide to ask the supervisors to appear at the Tribunal hearing.

ANNEX A

TO: C3 Division
     Home Office
     50 Queen Anne's Gate
     London SW1H 9AT

Report to the Home Secretary from the social supervisor of a conditionally discharged restricted patient

1. Patient's Name (Capitals).....................................

2. Home Office Reference number (if known) MNP/.....

3. Patient's Address...

    ....

4. Supervisor's Name..

5. Length of time since patient's conditional discharge

    ....

6. Frequency of meetings with the patient since last report

    ....

7. Does the patient show signs of becoming a danger to himself or others?

    ....

8. If the answer to 7 is Yes, what action does the supervisor recommend?

    ....

REPORT

(Please see paragraph 52 of the Home Office Notes for the guidance of social supervisors.)

Signed

Date

Line Manager's Comments (where appropriate)

Signed:

Date:

NB One copy of this report should be sent to the supervising psychiatrist and, for a period of about one year after discharge, two copies should be sent to the discharging hospital for the attention of the relevant clinical team.

ANNEX B

SUMMARY OF GUIDANCE ISSUED BY THE HOME OFFICE AND THE DEPARTMENT OF HEALTH TO SUPERVISING PSYCHIATRISTS

1. Staff in C3 Division of the Home Office are ready to discuss the case of any conditionally discharged patient with a supervising psychiatrist.
2. Prior to the conditional discharge of a patient the supervising psychiatrist should have an opportunity to get to know the patient and participate in at least one multidisciplinary case conference at the discharging hospital.
3. As early as possible prior to conditional discharge, a supervising psychiatrist should receive from the discharging hospital full written information about the patient's case (including the same information itemised in paragraph 26 of the Notes for the guidance of social supervisors).
4. A supervising psychiatrist is responsible for all matters relating to the mental health of the patient, including the regular assessment of the patient's condition, the monitoring of any necessary medication and the consideration of action in the event of deterioration in the patient's mental state.
5. The frequency and manner of psychiatric supervision and treatment appropriate in any case may be determined by the supervising psychiatrist.
6. The supervising psychiatrist should be prepared to be directly involved in the treatment and rehabilitation of the patient and to offer constructive support to the patient's progress in the community.
7. If a patient requires medication after discharge, then immediately after discharge, and again when any change or cessation of medication has been made, the supervising psychiatrist should inform the social supervisor and other members of the multidisciplinary team of the arrangements made, including when, where and by whom medication is to be given. Medication should also be one of the subjects covered in periodic discussions between a supervising psychiatrist and a social supervisor.
8. Close liaison between the supervising psychiatrist and the social supervisor is essential if supervision is to be effective and this should take the form of regular discussions.

Any clinical personnel involved with the patient should be under the general direction of the supervising psychiatrist.

9. The Home Office will usually ask a supervising psychiatrist for reports on the patient's progress one month after conditional discharge and every three months thereafter. The periodic report should include a detailed account of the patient's current mental condition, including any changes since the previous report and the apparent reasons for these changes. The report should always cover the subject of medication, where appropriate. Any signs of deterioration in the patient's mental health or behaviour should be described in detail, together with proposals for improving the situation. Finally, the report should include the supervising psychiatrist's plans for the patients continued rehabilitation.

10. All reports to the Home Office should be copied to the social supervisor. For about one year after discharge two copies of each report should also be sent to the hospital which discharged the patient.

11. Where a patient wishes to spend a holiday away from home and both supervisors agree to such a holiday, the supervising psychiatrist will wish to consider whether any special medication arrangements should be necessary.

12. Where a supervising psychiatrist is concerned about the conditionally discharged patient's mental state or behaviour, the concern should first be discussed, if possible, with the social supervisor. Where that concern amounts to a fear for the safety of the patient or of others, the supervising psychiatrist may decide to take immediate local action to admit the patient to hospital. Whether or not such action is taken, the supervising psychiatrist should report to the Home Office at once.

13. If a supervising psychiatrist considers that a patient no longer requires active psychiatric supervision, the matter should be discussed with the social supervisor and then an appropriate recommendation put forward to the Home Office. Where the Home Office agres to allow formal psychiatric supervision to lapse, it will usually wish social supervision to continue until it has seen evidence of a prolonged period of stability in the community.

14. A supervising psychiatrist is required, by the Tribunal Rules, to submit a report to a Mental Health Review Tribunal which is considering the case of a conditionally

discharged patient. The report, submitted via the Home Office, should include details of the patient's medical history, current mental state, response to psychiatric supervision and to any medication, and observations on the need for continuing psychiatric supervision.

ANNEX C

SUMMARY OF RECOMMENDATIONS FOR GOOD PRACTICE FOR STAFF OF THE DISCHARGING HOSPITAL

1. Preparation for discharge should begin as soon as such an outcome seems likely.
2. The multidisciplinary clinical team should instigate an individual programme of treatment and rehabilitation and reach a common view about the patient's expected approximate length of stay.
3. The hospital social work department should maintain links with outside individuals and agencies who may be able to offer support to the patient after discharge.
4. The multidisciplinary team should have a clear idea of the arrangements in the community which will best suit the patient.
5. The potential supervisors should be involved as early as practicable in the multidisciplinary team's preparations for the patient's discharge, with an opportunity to attend a case conference and meet the patient.
6. After the identification of supervision and after-care arrangements best suited to the patient's needs, nominated members of the multidisciplinary team should be responsible for arranging the various elements to be provided.
7. Where the choice of supervision between the probation service or the social services department is clearcut, a request for the nomination of an individual social supervisor, accompanied by information about the patient, should be made to the Chief Probation Officer or the Director of Social Services, as appropriate.
8. Where the choice of supervising agency is not clearcut or cannot be resolved quickly, information about the patient should be sent to both the Chief Probation Officer and the Director of Social Services with an invitation to send representatives to a case conference for discussion of the issue.
9. The responsible medical officer, after consultation with the other members of the multidisciplinary team, is responsible for arranging psychiatric supervision by a local consultant psychiatrist.

10. Responsibility for arranging suitable accommodation should be allocated by the multidisciplinary team to a named social worker or probation officer.
11. The views of the multidisciplinary team should be taken into account and the question of accommodation discussed in a pre-discharge case conference, attended by both supervisors.
12. It is important to identify suitable accommodation and to specify which types of accommodation would not be appropriate for individual patients.
13. There should be no question of a patient automatically going to unsuitable accommodation simply because a place is available and equal care is necessary whether the proposal for accommodation is to live with family or friends, or in lodgings or a hostel.
14. A member of staff of a proposed hostel should meet the patient and discuss the patient's needs with hospital staff.
15. The patient should visit and possibly spend a period of leave in a hostel before the decision is taken to accept an available place.
16. There are a number of important factors to be considered in the selection of a hostel for a particular patient.
17. The warden of the hostel should be given detailed information about the patient, including information which he may need about medication. He should be encouraged to contact the two supervisors and, if necessary, the social work department of the discharging hospital, for further information or advice.
18. Certain written information about the patient should be sent by the hospital social work department to supervising and after-care agencies on admission, as soon as discharge is in view and when nomination of a social supervisor is requested.
19. Supervisors should receive comprehensive, accurate and up-to-date information about a patient before he is discharged to their supervision. A standard package of information should be provided to both social and psychiatric supervisors as soon as they have been nominated.
20. Copies of supervisors' reports to the Home Office should be sent to the discharging hospital for a period of one year after discharge, for information.

21. After the conditional discharge of a patient, supervisors may sometimes seek information, guidance or support from those who know the patient well. It is hoped that discharging hospitals will be able to respond helpfully to such requests.

Glossary

(Extracted from D of H/HO (1992) *Review of Health and Social Services for Mentally Disordered Offenders and Others Requiring Similar Services*, (Reed Report), Cmnd 2088, HMSO, London.)

Reproduced by kind permission of C3 Division, Home Office.

Aggressive behaviour Verbal and/or physical actions or serious intentions that are outside the usually accepted range of harmful or confrontational behaviour, the consequences of which are likely to cause actual damage and/or real distress occurring either recently, persistently or with excessive severity.

Appropriate adult For the purposes of the Police and Criminal Evidence Act 1984:

(a) a relative, guardian or some other person responsible for the care or custody of a mentally disordered person;

(b) someone who has experience of dealing with mentally disordered people but is not a police officer or employed by the police;

(c) some other responsible adult aged 18 or over who is not a police officer or employed by the police (PACE Codes of Practice, Part C, Annex E).

Approved social worker A local social services authority has a duty under Section 114 of the Mental Health Act 1983 to appoint a sufficient number of approved social workers. A social worker who is approved must be experienced and have undertaken special training so that they have 'appropriate competence in dealing' with mentally disordered people.

Area committees Local committees, established in the light of the Woolf Report (Cm 1456, 1991) which bring together elements of the criminal justice system.

Assessment Active evaluation of needs. Can apply to individual needs for health or social care, or to the strategic assessment of service needs. See **Needs assessment** and **Risk assessment**.

Butler 1975 Report of the Committee on Mentally Abnormal Offenders (Cmnd 6244), chaired by the late Lord Butler of Saffron Walden.

Care Programme The 'Care Programme Approach' described in Health Circular (90)23/Local authority Letter (90)11 is designed 'to ensure that in future patients treated in the community receive the health and social care they need by:
(a) introducing more systematic arrangements for deciding whether a patient referred to the specialist psychiatric services can ... realistically be treated in the community;
(b) ensuring proper arrangements are then made and continue to be made, for the continuing health and social care of those patients who can be treated in the community.'

Central referral point A multi-agency referral point for mentally disordered offenders entering or moving between the health and social services.

Challenging behaviour Used in respect of people with learning disabilities or other mental disorders who exhibit behavioural disturbance through assaultive, aggressive or destructive and/or irresponsible behaviour.

Circular 66/90 Home Office circular of 3 September 1990 on provision for mentally disordered offenders.

Clinical Relating to professional aspects of health care work.

Codes of Practice
(a) Mental Health Act. Prepared under Section 18 of the Mental Health Act 1983. It provides detailed guidance on how the provisions of the Mental Health Act 1983 should be operated.
(b) PACE. Prepared under Section 66 of the Police and Criminal Evidence Act 1984, Code C. Annex E summarizes provisions relating to mentally disordered people.

Care team Local multiprofessional teams responsible for 'ensuring that mentally disordered offenders within a defined area are properly assessed at the "point of entry" (and as necessary thereafter) and then receive, or are referred to those who will provide the continuing care and treatment they need in the right kind of setting'. The assessment panel schemes that have been established in some areas fulfil a similar, though more limited, function.

Courts In England and Wales there are 511 magistrates courts and 87 Crown Courts. The powers of magistrates courts to try and to sentence are limited to summary offences only. More serious cases are dealt with by the Crown Court.

Court assessment and diversion schemes See **Diversion**.

Dangerousness The difficulty in defining the concept of 'dangerousness' was addressed in depth by the Butler Committee (Cmnd 6244, 1975). For its own purposes, the Committee equate it 'to a potential for acts which are likely to cause serious physical or lasting psychological harm'. But considerable reservations have been expressed about this and, indeed, about most other attempts at definitive statements of what 'dangerousness' entails. It is evident that there are widely varying forms and levels of dangerousness as regards both the clinical condition of the individual concerned and the circumstances in which the individual finds himself at any particular time. But the issue of dangerousness, and of the means of assessing and predicting its incidence in individual cases in a consistent and objective way, is central to the work of forensic psychiatry.

Differing needs See **Special differing needs**.

Difficult to place Applied to people with a recognized mental disorder which results in their displaying at times unacceptable and/or disturbed behaviour which requires specialist assessment, treatment, rehabilitation and care in a flexible (non-permanently) secure environment. Such patients may have previously demonstrated an inability to benefit from provision by the acute psychiatric services as a result of exhibiting behaviour which requires treatment in a more structured and controlled environment over a period greater than that required to deal with an acute psychiatric emergency. Such people often require multi-agency involvement in their care or services which may not always be readily available.

Discontinuance When the Crown Prosecution Service decides not to proceed with a criminal prosecution.

District Health Authority One of more than 180 statutory bodies in England which are responsible for ensuring the purchase of health care for their resident population.

Diversion Enabling a mentally disordered offender (or alleged offender) to receive care and treatment from services other than those provided by the criminal justice system. In practice, the term is most often applied when this happens at or just before a court appearance but could also apply to diverting people from police stations or remand prisons. There is a growing number and range of course assessment and diversion schemes to identify individual needs and advise as to suitable disposals.

Duty psychiatrist scheme A type of court assessment and diversion scheme (see **Diversion**).

Emergency application Admission for assessment in cases of emergency under Section 4 of the Mental Health Act 1983. In exceptional cases it may be necessary to admit a person for assessment as an emergency without obtaining a second medical recommendation. An emergency application may be made by an approved social worker or by a person's nearest relative. It must state that it is of urgent necessity for the person to be admitted to hospital and detained for assessment, and that compliance with the normal procedures would involve undesirable delay.

Family Health Services Authority FHSAs are responsible for managing the services provided under the NHS by family doctors, dentists, community pharmacists and ophthalmic opticians. FHSAs are accountable to Regional Health Authorities and work in close collaboration with district health authorities.

Forensic psychiatry Forensic means pertaining to, or connected with, or used in the course of law. A forensic psychiatrist's work may be said to start with the preparation of psychiatric reports for the court on the mental state of offenders suspected of having a mental abnormality. The psychiatrist will then be expected to provide or arrange treatment for the mentally (disordered) offender where appropriate. Other psychiatrists and other professionals seeing the sort of patient the forensic psychiatrist is looking after will refer similar patients who may not actually have reached the court or broken the law. In practice all psychiatrists may, at some time or another, have to prepare psychiatric reports on their own patients. Some general psychiatrists have a special interest or responsibility in forensic psychiatry. The term 'forensic psychiatry' is used to describe those for whom this is their principal work' (Faulk (1988) *Basic Forensic Psychiatry*).

Glancy 1974 Report of the Department of Health and Social Security Working party on Security in NHS Psychiatric Hospitals, chaired by Dr J.E. Glancy. The 'Glancy Target' for medium secure psychiatric provision was based on an estimate of 20 beds per million population.

Health Care Service for Prisoners Formerly the Prison Medical Service. This is the part of the prison service responsible for the delivery of health care to prisoners. Following the 1990 Efficiency Scrutiny it will become a 'purchaser' rather than a 'provider'.

High security see **Security (high)**.

'Interim' Secure Unit A psychiatric facility established pending the development of a permanent regional Secure Uit which provides treatment in law to medium security.

Irresponsible Conduct, behaviour or real intentions that show a serious disregard for the consequences of the actions taken and where the results cause actual damage or real distress either recently or persistently or with excessive severity to self or others.

Learning difficulties Educational needs requiring special educational provision within the meaning of the Education Act 1981. Distinct from 'learning disabilities' (see below), but has nevertheless been used by some as a synonym for 'mental handicap'.

Learning disabilities Term adopted for 'mental handicap'. Applies to people with a state of arrested or incomplete development of mind which includes significant disabilities of intelligence and social functioning. Includes mentally impaired and severely mentally impaired people within the terms of the Mental Health Act 1983.

Local authority The council of a county, a metropolitan district or a London borough or the Common Council of the City of London.

Medium secure units see **Security (medium)**.

Mental disorder

(a) Legal term, pertaining to the Mental Health Act 1983, Section 1(2):

mental disorder means mental illness, arrested or incomplete development of mind, psychopathic disorder and any other disorder or disability of mind and 'mentally disordered' shall be construed accordingly;

severe mental impairment means a state of arrested or incomplete development of mind which includes severe impairment of intelligence and social functioning and is associated with abnormally aggressive or irresponsible conduct on the part of the person concerned and 'severely mentally impaired' shall be construed accordingly;

mental impairment means a state of arrested or incomplete development of mind (not amounting to severe mental impairment) which includes significant impairment of intelligence and social functioning and is associated with abnormally aggressive conduct on the part of the person concerned and 'mentally impaired' shall be construed accordingly;

psychopathic disorder means a persistent disorder or disability of mind (whether or not including significant impairment of intelligence) which results in abnormally aggressive or seriously irresponsible conduct on the part of the person concerned.

(b) also a collective term of the World Health Organisation classification of diseases relating to mental ill health.

mentally disordered offender A mentally disordered person who has broken the law. In identifying broad service needs, this term is sometimes loosely used to include mentally disordered people who are alleged to have broken the law.

Mental handicap See **Learning disabilities**.

Mental Health Act Mental Health Act 1983.

Mental impairment: See **Mental disorder**.

Mental illness A disturbance of thought, mood, volition, perception, orientation or memory which impairs judgement or behaviour to a significant extent.

Multi-agency group In terms of mentally disordered offenders, a local group that brings together elements of the health, social and criminal justice services, and other services as necessary.

Needs

(a) '**The need for health** is a broad term typically measured by health questions in health surveys, surrogate measures such as deprivation indices, and relative measures such as standardised mortality ratios – all measures which do not easily translate into what can or should be done to improve health' (NHS Management Executive (1991) *Assessing Health Care Needs*).

(b) '**The need for health care** is much more specific. It is dependent on the availability or potential availability of health care and prevention services to respond to the disease or risk factors – and to secure an improvement in health, i.e. the ability to benefit from effective health care or prevention services' (NHS Management Executive (1991) *Assessing Health Care Needs*).

(c) **Social care needs** 'Social services departments should identify the care needs of the local population taking into account factors such as age distribution, problems associated with living in inner-city areas or rural areas, special needs of ethnic minority communities, the number of homeless or transient people likely to need care. From April 1993 plans should identify client groups for whom services are to be arranged, how care needs of individuals will be assessed and how identified service needs will be incorporated into the planning process. The interface between health care and social care is a key area. Concerned authorities should establish shared appreciation of how local needs should be delivered' (*Community Care in the Next Decade and Beyond*).

Needs assessment A means of defining the nature and level of services required to care for and improve the health of a population (see NHS Management Executive (1991) *Assessing Health Care Needs*). An initial framework for assessing the service needs of mentally disordered offenders was set out in Management Executive Letter (92)24.

Outreach services These are all the activities of agencies relating to a service for mentally disordered offenders which are additional to in-patient assessment, treatment, rehabilitation and after-care of patients. They are community-based resources, often to be found in major conurbations and include such developments as out-patient departments, daycentres, drop-in centres, sheltered hostels and housing.

PACE Police and Criminal Evidence Act 1984.

Panel scheme An extended form of **court assessment and diversion scheme** (see **Care Team** and **Diversion**).

Police There are 43 police forces in England and Wales. Their main functions in relation to mentally disordered offenders are set out in Home Office Circular 66/90, paragraph 4.

Prisons There are about 130 prisons in England and Wales grouped into 15 areas. The prison service's main obligations are: to implement the court's decision by keeping the prisoner in custody; to provide a positive regime to help the prisoner make the best use of the time in prison; and to prepare the prisoner for release (see *Custody, Care and Justice*, Cm 1647, paragraphs 1.22–1.28). Wherever possible, mentally disordered offenders should receive care and treatment from health and social services rather than in custodial care.

Prison Medical Service See **Health Care Service for Prisoners**.

Probation Service There are 55 Probation Service areas in England and Wales which mostly correspond to county boundaries. The special role of the probation service is:

- to provide information to the courts for bail and sentencing decisions;
- to provide information to the Crown Prosecution Service in connection with bail information schemes;
- to provide bail and probation hostels and other accommodation projects for offenders and persons on bail;
- to supervise offenders on probation orders;
- to provide for the throughcare and supervision of offenders released from prison on licence and parole (Home Office Circular 66/90).

Provider Any person, group of persons, organizations, facilities or units supplying health or social services.

Psychopathic disorder See **Mental disorder**.

Purchaser/Commissioner A person or body who buys services, including GP fundholders, health and local authorities.

Reed Department of Health/Home Office review of services for mentally disordered offenders and others requiring similar services (1991–2), the Steering committee of which was chaired by Dr John Reed (Senior Principal Medical Officer, DH).

Regional Health Authority One of the 14 statutory bodies in England which are responsible for overseeing the work of a number of District Health Authorities.

Regional Secure Unit See **Security (medium)**.

Restriction Order An order applied by a Crown Court, in addition to a hospital order under the Mental Health Act 1983, which reserves power to the Home Secretary to restrict leave of absence, and transfer or discharge and a Mental Health Review Tribunal to discharge or grant leave of absence.

Risk assessment 'Risk may be viewed not only in terms of possible physical harm to others or to the patient himself. It may include such eventualities as distress or embarrassment, damage to property, or other offending. It is important that, wherever possible, assessments of risk . . . are undertaken on a multidisciplinary basis'.

Screening An initial examination to determine whether there are any symptoms which could point to mental disorder. Such an indication should lead to a referral for a medical assessment.

Security

(a) **Low**: Some local hospitals have wards coping with 'difficult' patients which provide a degree of physical security by being locked or having an above-average staff ratio. These are sometimes known as 'intensive care units'.

(b) **Medium**: Units (including regional Secure Units) which care for patients who are too difficult or dangerous for local hospitals but who do not require the higher security available at Special Hospitals.

(c) **High**: Provided in Special Hospitals under the aegis of the Special Hospitals Service Authority. They provide a similar range of therapeutic services as ordinary psychiatric hospitals but in a level of utmost security to enable the treatment of patients detained under the Mental Health Act and who, in the opinion of the Secretary of State, require this because of their dangerousness, violent or criminal propensities. The regimes of care and observation are such that can only be justified when a high level of security is required and a lesser degree of security would not provide a reasonable safeguard to the public.

Serious Important and demanding consideration.

Severe Violent, extreme, making great demands upon.

Smith formula Method used by the Department of Health for calculating enhanced revenue funding for Health Regions that achieve two-thirds of their bed target for medium secure psychiatric provision. (It is named after the official who devised it.)

Social Services Authority The council of a non-metropolitan country, metropolitan district, London borough, or the Common Council of the City of London.

Social Services Department The department of the social services authority headed by the Director of Social Services Departments.

Special Hospital See **Security (High)**.

Special Hospitals Service Authority the SHSA was established in 1989 to manage the three Special Hospitals:

Ashworth in Merseyside, Rampton in Nottinghamshire and Broadmoor in Berkshire. The hospitals were previously managed directly by the Department of Health. They care for patients requiring treatment under conditions of special security: see **Security (High)**.

Special/differing needs 'Special needs group is a term of convenience. It serves to identify certain individual patients whose needs are similar and specialised enough to present **special issues** for those purchasing and providing services' (SN 2.1). The term **differing needs** is increasingly preferred to 'special' needs.

Treatability When medical treatment is considered likely to alleviate or prevent a deterioration of a person's condition.

Treatment Professional responses aimed at reducing or removing the signs and symptoms of the mental disorder suffered by the patient and including nursing care, habilitation and rehabilitation.

Trust A hospital trust is a legal body within the NHS which has the power and responsibility to govern a hospital or group of hospitals.

Woolf 1991 report (Cm 1456) of an inquiry by Lord Justice Woolf into prison disturbances that occurred in April 1990. A number of its recommendations were adopted in the White Paper *Custody, Care and Justice* (Cm 1647).

Woolf committees See **Area committees**.

Index

Aarvold Board 147
  see also Aarvold Report
Aarvold Report 140-1, 146,
    147, 154
Access to services
  cultural and linguistic 8
Admission to special hospital
  relevant legislation 142
  role of social worker 142-4
Aggression 79-98
  anticipation of 95
  in daycare settings 96-7
  on home visits 95-6
  interview method 97
  in office settings 96
  physical intervention 98
  in residential settings 96-7
  and transporting clients 98
Alcohol and drug dependency
    4
American Medical Inc 195
Appropriate adult 39, 120-4
  appointment of 122-3
  choice of 121-3
  police interview 123-4
  referral 121-3
  at the police station 123-4
  see also Police and Criminal
      Evidence Act 1984
Approved social worker 69-70,
    71
Ashworth Hospital 28, 140,
    141-2
  enquiry 141-2

social work department
    141-2
  see also Special hospital
      system
Assessment 17-19
Assertiveness 17
Attempted suicide, *see* Suicide
Attitudes 13-15
  see also Values
Authority, use of 80, 90

Bethlem Hospital 24
Black
  definitions of 52-3
  history 72
  hostels 53
  issues in residential and
      daycare settings 67, 72
  mentally disordered
      offenders 15
Bow St. and Marlborough St.
    Magistrates Court Panel
    Assessment Scheme 118-19
Bridewell 23
Broadmoor Hospital 24, 28,
    140, 141
  see also Special hospital
      system
Butler Committee 30
  final report 1975 30
  interim report 1974 30

C3 Division, Home Office, *see*
    Home Office

Campbell, Sharon 10, 93
Care management 40, 70, 108, 124–6
Care manager, *see* Care management
Care programme approach 34–5, 44, 126, 134–5
 role of keyworker 134, 136
Carstairs hospital 140
Case management, *see* Care management
Chlorpromazine group of drugs 25
Clunis, Christopher 93, 136, 176, 188, 198
Collaboration, *see* Joint planning/working
Community care 13, 23, 29, 39–40, 171, 195–8
Community Mental Health Centre Act 1963 (USA) 40
Community psychiatric nurses 59, 111
 training 200–1
Community Supervision Order (proposed) 44–5
Confidentiality 64
County Asylums Act 1808 24
Criminal Justice Act 1972 43
Criminal Justice Act 1991 42–3
Criminal Lunatics Act 1800 23, 24
Criminal Lunatics Act 1860 24
Criminal Procedure (Insanity and Unfitness to Plead) Act 1991 41–2
 absolute discharge 42
 disposal options 41
 guardianship order 41
 hospital order 41
 medical evidence 41
 supervision and treatment order 41, 130–1
 a trial of facts 41
Crown Court 32
Crown Prosecution Service 32
Custodial care 23

Dangerousness 10, 79–98, 182
 in the community 79–80
 in institutional settings 79
Daycare
 communication 189–93
 discharge from 188–9
 ethnicity issues 185
 ethos 185–6
 referrals 182–3
 tasks and functions 178–9
 teamwork 179
Defining the mentally disordered offender 6–12
Deliberate self harm, *see* Suicide
Department of Health
 management of special hospitals 28
Depression 7, 31, 74–5, 84
Disadvantage 2
 see also Inequality
Discharge from special hospital 146–50
Disclosure of information 160–1
Discrimination 2–5, 48–78
 combatting 63
 definition of 49–51
 ethnicity and 52–3
 indirect 50–1
 racial 52–3, 64–72
 sexual 53, 72–6
 and staff stress 77
Distinctive way of working 12–20
Diversion from custody 10, 15, 31–2, 108, 114–18
 and the courts 32
 and the Crown Prosecution Service 32
 funding of 32
 Hull project 115–18
 and the police 31
Diversion to treatment, *see* Diversion from custody
Duty to warn 111

Empathy 16–17
Employment 160

Ethnic monitoring
  in residential work 182
Ethnicity 52-3
  and race 184-5
Ethnic minorities
  and the Reed Report 33
Ethnic sensitivity 53, 184-5

Families 143-6, 148
Female mentally disordered
    offenders, *see* Mentally
    disordered offenders,
    female
Forensic psychiatry 35
Forensic social work, *see* Social
  work

George III 24
Glancy Report 1974 30
Gordon, Paul 3-4
Grendon Underwood prison 27
Guardianship 41, 44, 131-4
  see also Criminal Justice
      Act 1991; Criminal
      Procedures (Insanity
      and Unfitness to Plead)
      Act 1991; Mental
      Health Act 1983
Hadfield, James 24
Health of the Nation 203-4
Health service
  changes in 172
Hertfordshire Panel Assessment
    Scheme 119, 129
Historical background 23-5
Home Office 153, 157, 161, 163
Home Office Circular 66/90
    31-2, 115
Home visiting 17
Horsley, William 3
Hostels 148, 150
  admission contract for 174
  black 53
  black advisory group 184-5
  black staff 184
  communication in 189-93
  discharge from 187-8
  discrimination in 50-1
  ethos of 183-5

management of 174
mental health 174, 178
and placement breakdown
    187
power in 54-5
primary task of 174-6
probation 51, 174, 177, 179
referrals 179-82
staff attitudes 62
see also Residential and
    daycare services;
    Residential work
Hull diversion from custody
    project 115-18
see also Diversion from
    custody
Human volcano 79-85

Inter-agency working, *see* Joint
    planning/working
Indefinite detention 24
Inequality 48
  see also Disadvantage
Inter-agency co-operation
  and diversion 32, 33-4
  and probation orders with a
      condition of psychiatric
      treatment 43-4, 129
  see also Joint planning/
      working; Inter-
      professional working
Interim Secure Units 11
Interpreters 70-1
Interprofessional working
  case conferences 189
Intrusive style of working
    17-19, 56
  supervision of staff 157-61,
      201-3
Invisible mentally disordered
    offenders 6-8

Jansen, Elly 183
Joint management, *see* Joint
    planning/working
Joint planning/working 203-6
  hybrid agency 205
  see also Inter-agency
      co-operation

Kneesworth Hospital 195–6, 203

Legislation relevant to mentally disordered offenders 36–45
Local hospitals 25–6
Locked wards 25–6
    and Reed Report 26
    see also Open door movement
Lunatics Act 1845 24

Magistrates Court 32
Management support 201–3
Medical model 4–5
Mental Deficiency Act 1913 24
Mental disorder and offending behaviour 8
Mental Health Act 1959 25, 28, 141
Mental Health Act 1983 28, 36–8, 113, 149–50, 152
Mental Health Act Commission
    recommendations for transfer and discharge arrangements 147
Mental Health Act Review Tribunals 147, 165, 167
    transfer and discharge from special hospitals 147
Mentally disordered offenders
    black 15, 52–3, 64–72
    definition of 6–12
    female 5–7, 72–6
    incidence 6–12
    invisible 6–8, 107
    older 7
    recognized 6, 11–12
Mental Treatment Act 1930 24
Miller, E. and Gwynne, M. 174–6, 183
Monitoring
    in daycare 178–9, 182
    in residential care 177–8
Moss Side hospital 24, 28
    see also Special hospital system

Mother and baby units
    in Regional Secure Units 73–4
Mudd, Daniel 76, 160, 162–3, 181
Murder followed by suicide 99

NACRO 32
National Health Service and Community Care Act 1990 32, 39–40, 203
Non-intervention 14

Offenders
    with mental health needs 6, 8–10
Open door movement 25, 26, 28, 29
    see also Locked wards

Park Lane Hospital 28
    see also Special hospital system
Partnership with the client 13
Patients
    who offend 6, 8–11
Personality disorder 4, 81, 84, 101, 135
Police 31–2
Police and Criminal Evidence Act 1984 (Section 66) 38–9
Power 13–15, 54
    of the client 56–7
    in fieldwork 56
    in hostels 54–5
    inequality in 13
    in prisons and hospitals 55
    statutory 54, 56, 57
Powers of Criminal Courts Act 1973 43
Pownall, Judge 3
Prejudice 2, 49–52, 57, 60–1
    against mentally disordered offenders 49–52, 57–9, 172
    see also Discrimination; Inequality; Stigma

Prevention 107–9
primary 112–14
secondary 107, 109–12
tertiary 107
Prison health care system 115
Prison Medical Service 27–8, 32
Prison population 9
remand 9–10, 27
sentenced 10, 27
Prison system 26–8, 108–9
and Judge Tumin 109
Private hospitals 195–6
American Medical International Inc 195
Kneesworth House Hospital 195–6, 203
St Andrews Hospital, Northampton 195
Stockton Hall Hospital 195
Probation hostels 61–2, 174, 179–80
Probation officers 62, 65, 111, 146, 152
training of 199–201
Probation order with a condition of psychiatric treatment 9, 43–4, 126–30
and inter-agency working 129, 134
Probation service 9, 13, 15, 32, 172
Psychiatric nursing 15, 59, 111
training 200–1
Psychiatric Panel Assessment Schemes 118–20
Bow St. and Marlborough St. Magistrates Court 118–19
Hertfordshire 119, 129
Psychopathic disorder, *see* Personality disorder

Race 52–3
and ethnicity 184–5
Racism
and British culture 68–9, 71–2
and Hitler 67–8
and language 71–2
Rampton Hospital 24, 28, 140
see also Special hospital system
Recognized mentally disordered offenders 6, 11–12
Recording 18
Reed Committee, *see* Reed Report
Reed Report 26, 33–4, 115, 130
and ethnic minority groups 33, 50, 64–7
and locked wards 26
and women 33
Regional Secure Units 11, 29–31
and mother and baby units 73–4
Register of potentially violent patients 111, 189
Relationship building 16
Residential and daycare services 173–8
and black service users 67, 72
Residential work 7
admission contract 174
communication in 189–93
discharge from 187–8
ethnicity in 184
ethnic monitoring 182
ethos of 183–5
the 'horticultural' model 174–6
hostels 173
leadership 191–3
maintenance function 176
management 176
the primary task 174–6
tasks and functions of 173–8
teamwork 189, 193
the 'warehousing model' 174–6
Revolving door 11
Richmond Fellowship 183
Risk
assessing 157–60
to the client 93–104

Risk *contd*
 to others 85–91, 160
 to the public 60
 to the worker 80–2, 91–8,
  159

Safety 10
Sandwell Metropolitan
  Borough 69–70
Schizophrenia 3, 4, 8, 81, 85
Schwarz, Isobel 10, 93
Section 117 149–50
Secure provision
 erosion of 195
Silcock, Ben 198
Social supervision of the
  restricted patient in the
  community
 and C3 Division, Home
  Office 153, 157, 161,
  163
 change of supervisor 162–3
 dilemmas 157–61
 disclosure of information
  160–1
 intrusive style of 158–60
 numbers under 150
 preparation for 151–4
 the process of 154–7
 recall from 163–5
 teamwork in 161–2
 termination of 165–7
Social work 111, 140–50
 in psychiatric hospitals 140
 in Regional Secure Units
  142
 in special hospitals 140–50
 training for 199–201
Sociopathic disorder, *see*
  Personality disorder
Special Hospitals Service
  Authority 28–9
Special hospital system 11,
  28–9, 140–50
 admission to 142–4
 Ashworth 28, 140, 141–2
 Broadmoor 24, 28, 140, 141
 Carstairs 140
 discharge from 140, 146–50

Moss Side 24, 28
Park Lane 28
Rampton 24, 28, 140
 social work in 140–50
 throughcare 144–6
St Andrews Hospital 195
Staff
 untrained 171, 189
 see also Training
Staff supervision, *see*
  Supervision of the
  worker
Stigma 8, 11, 20, 29, 109
 see also Discrimination;
  Prejudice
Suicide 18–19, 98–104, 135
 attempted 18–19
 intervention 100–4
 in prison 99
Supervised discharge
  arrangements (proposed)
  44–5
Supervision of the client
 intrusive style of 17–19
 knowledge for 15–16
 skills needed for 16–20
 see also Social supervision
Supervision of the worker 17,
  61–2, 167–8, 202–3
 using intrusive style of client
  supervision 201–3
 management support 200–3
Supervision Register 35, 135–6

Tarasoff ruling 111
Throughcare in special
  hospitals 144–6
 length of stay 144
 role of social worker 145–6
Toronto Forensic Service 8–9
Training 198–201
 of approved social workers
  200
 CCETSW report on 199
 of hostel and daycare staff 201
 of psychiatric nurses 200–1
 the Reed Report 199
 of social workers 199–201
 of probation officers 199–201

Transfer and discharge from
    special hospital 146–50
  choice of hostel 148–50
  Mental Health Act Review
    Tribunal 146
  recommendation of the
    Home Secretary 146–7
  role of social worker 148
Treatability 4–5
Trial of Lunatics Act 1883 41

Unitary authorities 172

Vagrancy Act 1714 23
Vagrancy Act 1744 23
Values 13–15
  see also Attitudes

Violence
  domestic 112
  duty to warn 111
  and powerlessness 80
  and psychosis 81, 84, 85
  Tarasoff ruling 111
  see also Aggression
Voluntary treatment 24
Volunteers 171
  black 185

Women
  and the Reed Report 33

Young, Graham 140, 159

Zito, Jonathan 93, 198